CONSENT:
PRACTICAL PRINCIPLES FOR CLINICIANS

BY

Jeffrey C. McILwain

eBooks End User License Agreement

DEDICATION

To Nick Whalley partner and friend

CONTENTS

CHAPTERS

ABOUT THE AUTHOR

Jeff McIlwain is a Consultant, Clinical Risk Management in a NHS Teaching Hospitals Trust in the North West of the U.K. He was trained in Northern Ireland at Queens University Belfast and rotated through the Northern Ireland training programme in ENT surgery. He was the Conacher Fellow at the University of Toronto in 1986 and worked in basic science research of the posterior glottis. From this work he was awarded his Doctorate in Medicine (MD) from Queens University Belfast in 1988. This was one of the first MDs in the speciality in the UK. He was appointed as ENT consultant and Clinical Director to the Trust in 1991 and developed the unit to be the best regionally for its size at that time. From 1996 he has been involved in Clinical Risk Management and published 26 clinical and 17 clinical risk papers and given over 100 lectures.

FOREWORD

Correct and up to date knowledge of consent for clinical care is fundamental to good clinical practice and patient communication. Most clinicians in busy wards and clinics will recognize that there is considerable room for improvement in seeking and recording consent at present from most patients in such locations. Furthermore, as case law on consent has evolved significantly over recent years as has guidance from the Department of Health and General Medical Council, the need for concise practical up to date guidance for front line staff is palpable. It thus gives me great pleasure to introduce this topical guide *Consent, Practical Principles for Clinicians* by Mr. Jeffrey McIlwain. It will be of use to clinicians, risk managers and lawyers. The clarity of presentation, in what is often a difficult subject for many of us, is especially appealing. While this short book is modestly presented as a broad overview to consent in clinical practice, it covers the subject matter comprehensively. For those who like to know that little bit more, the text is thoroughly referenced. While the context principally relates to English law and current clinical practice in the UK it will be also of interest to international readers in jurisdictions that often draw upon such principles.

Jeff McIlwain is ideally placed to present such a guide to healthcare professionals given his dual surgical and clinical risk expertise and experience. The author's approach to this subject is both conceptual and practical and is aptly illustrated with clinical and legal cases examples. A final 'stretch yourself' self test section provides numerous scenarios that will exercise healthcare practitioners' key knowledge and skills in consent. Consideration of these scenarios will also be a bonus to medical practitioners presenting for Appraisal and for those seeking Revalidation as well as being an educational bonus for clinical training.

If I may speak directly to those undertaking consent for treatment; you can be grateful that there is a handy book such as this as an aid to navigation in this field. This is a key item to buy and read now and to then return when uncertain waters reappear, as they will do. The clinician aiming for best practice on consent will keep this textbook close at hand and will re-visit it as a reference when new clinical challenges in consent are encountered.

SIMON P KELLY *FRCSEd, FRCOphth, FEBO*
Consultant Ophthalmic Surgeon,
Bolton, England

PREFACE

This book is a reflection of working in the field of consent for a decade by the author. The text takes a broad view of consent in healthcare rather than a large in depth review of large textbook / reference books. The aim is to give less experienced clinicians this broad overview with some depth around clinical consent to hopefully stimulate readers to explore deeper. There may indeed be errors within the text which are entirely the authors. There may also be differing views on interpreting some of the opinion. If this is the case I apologise, however, to ford the breadth rather than investigate the depth does mean that some detail or interpretation must be sacrificed. Nevertheless I hope that what is found within will be of value. No doubt those of a pedantic disposition will be dismayed by the use of hard and soft words and possibly quibble of the meaning of some expressions and their interpretation, however, the text should be viewed as an entity rather than a collection of erudite essays and it is the overall meaning that is important rather than intricate specifics.

Many references reflect the era we now live in i.e. the use of the World Wide Web and so further referencing texts will point to such web sites. To some there may be a paucity of references. Those references selected are for illustrative or factual purposes or as a resource to follow. Most are as contemporaneous as possible. The author has avoided digest of opinion as that would mean that there is a presumption the author has read and understood all the texts rather than inadvertently citing references to demonstrate a provenance. Further for every opinion of 'yea' there is often a body of opinion of 'nay'. The aims of the text and references are to show basic principles for clinical practice rather than digest of opinion or furnish the ultimate bibliography of all that has been written.

Jeffrey C. McILwain
St. Helens & Knowsley Teaching Hospitals
UK

BACKGROUND TO THE TEXT

To most people within healthcare, consent is largely taken to mean a legal obligation and the consequent legal ramifications. However this puts aside the elements and principles of clinical ethics and the more recent development of Clinical Risk Management input to the end solution. A legal consultation may result in advice and decision 'A' but set against an ethics and or clinical risk management opinion in a more collaborative opinion a differing decision or opinion may result i.e. decision 'B'. To use a singular discipline to ascertain the correct or just answer to a consent issue is inherently risky, however, by intertwining clinical law, ethics and risk management a more balanced and just decision may be made. The purpose of this book is to try to blend basic clinical law, ethics and risk management to help clinicians formulate a just decision yet set against the boundaries of each discipline.

At the core of consent is the right, owned by the patient, to donate their authority to another person to allow the second person to touch them. In the clinical area this reflects a patient presenting to a clinician for advice and treatment management. When a patient enters into a consultation there is no *de facto* right for the clinician to presume to proceed just because the patient is there within the clinician's environment. There is an axiom in risk management – "Never presume". In the matter of consent never presume that the patient being volitionally present equates to an agreement or a granting of permission to the clinician to go further and perform an invasive clinical procedure without seeking the authority to do so from the patient.

The setting and context of the book is centred on the National Health Service (NHS) of England and Wales. Within the UK there are differences in principles, particularly in law in the different component countries. For example in Scotland the age of majority in consent is taken as age 16 rather than 18 or 16 as it is in other parts of the UK [1]. The age of majority changed on 1st January 1970 from age 21 to age 18 in England and 16 in Scotland. However, the purpose of this book is less about differing local detail which a Healthcare Professional should check on and more about generic or encompassing principles. Equally the principles may apply to other countries.

A few decades ago this type of book would be pointed towards doctors and lawyers in medico-legal practice. Recent changes in the professional workforce and within the UK and NHS healthcare delivery system resulted in a substantial shift both in the importance of consent and also to the skills that Healthcare Professionals must now have. The traditional demarcation between a doctor's role and a nurse's role has changed and many nurses now perform procedures that were previously or traditionally the sole province of doctors. Further still, certain procedures that nurses performed have become the skill role of Health Care Assistants and others such as Operating Department Assistants. As well there has been a rise in the role of autonomous independent practitioners in nursing who have achieved a level of competence that matches or even supersedes that of a doctor in training. Other developments today and in the future include moving clinical procedures from the traditional secondary care sector to the primary care sector. Yet, the procedures themselves require the same context of consent irrespective of whoever performs the procedure or advises upon it, or where it is done. There is a decanting downwards of more basic skills and attendant procedures from one professional group to another and to other professional groups. The clinical interface between a patient and a professional may change but consent remains the same.

REFERENCE

[1]   HM Revenue & Customs. Manuals. Decision Makers Guide DMG 47063
http://www.hmrc.gov.uk/manuals/dmgmanual/html/DMG46001/10_0092_DMG47063.htm

INTRODUCTION

Consent is a fundamental principle that shapes the relationship between a patient and a clinician. A clinician cannot proceed to deliver, in physical terms, the proposed system of healthcare management for a disease or a disorder without the patient giving their permission to do so. Over the past century there has been a shift from medical paternalism of "I know what is best for you and you shall have it" towards a more autonomous approach of "Please make up your mind of what is best for you". This process has accelerated over the past 15 years largely due to the effects of the litigation process. Prior to 1991 in the UK doctors subscribed to Medical Defence Organisations (MDOs) to protect themselves from allegations of clinical negligence. The NHS effectively devolved such negligence issues to be part of the professional's life. Crown Immunity [1, 2] protected NHS employees from prosecution of a criminal matter. When this was lifted within the NHS in 1990 it was replaced by Crown Indemnity [3] whereby each NHS organisation became directly responsible for the acts of its employees, including allegations of negligence. Thereafter the establishment of the NHS Litigation Authority (NHSLA) to manage and monitor allegations of negligence resulted in recognition of the need for stronger risk management controls within NHS organisations and so the concept of the Clinical Negligence Scheme for Trusts (CNST) was born whereby there would be standardised risk imperatives to be achieved [4].

Part of these standards includes consent and this stimulated the UK Department of Health to produce standardised consent forms and guidance [5, 6] in 2003 throughout the NHS. Organisations within the NHS who wish to achieve a reduction in their contribution to the mutuality of the crown indemnity provided through NHSLA must subscribe to these standardised forms.

Part of the acceleration of consent taking and giving has been realised through events in Alder Hey Hospital *vis a vis* organ retention with the establishment of the Human Tissue Authority in 2004 [7] to cover the donation, storage and display of human tissue for various purposes. The fields of medical research which already had a strong consent position have also been strengthened [8] within the UK Medical Research Council (MRC).

It is apparent that faced with a change from immunity to indemnity and a rising ability of the legal profession within the area of negligence that consent has risen from "sign this piece of paper" to a complicated system with internal auditing through risk management processes and evidence trails.

That there is a less than 100% ability or compliance in consent has been shown in a survey published by Hamilton [9] whereby the range of ability to obtain complete "informed consent" between FY 1&2, SpR and Consultant surgeons varied between 69% and 80%. In obtaining consent from children this varied between 50% and 64%, from psychiatric patients between 70% and 90% and for research and screening between 80% and 100%. Although this was a small sample and a survey it rather defies the belief that consent taking has actually penetrated the professional surgeon's training and ability even in 2007. Interestingly the SpR group (registrars) fared best overall suggesting that senior trainees better more junior trainees and even their peers and trainers!

REFERENCES

[1] Select Committee on Public Accounts Minutes of Evidence APPENDIX 2 Supplementary memorandum submitted by HM Treasury http://www.publications.parliament.uk/pa/cm200203/cmselect/cmpubacc/ 588/2102314 .htm

[2] Public and Commercial Services Union Knowledge Centres / Health and Safety / Legal Summaries / Crown Immunity http://www.pcs.org.uk/Templates/Internal.asp?NodeID=884239

[3] bma.org.uk Archive/Archive - Medical careers and education Guide for doctors new to the UK October 2004 http://www.bma.org.uk/ap.nsf/Content/GuidefordoctorsnewtoUK~indemnity

[4] NHS Litigation Authority Clinical Negligence Scheme for Trusts (CNST) http://www.nhsla.com/Claims/Schemes/CNST/

[5] Department of Health Policy and Guidance about the consent form http://www.dh.gov.uk/en/Policyandguidance/Healthandsocialcaretopics/Consent/Consentgeneralinformation/DH_4015937

[6] Department of Health Policy and Guidance consent key documents http://www.dh.gov.uk/en/Policyandguidance/Healthandsocialcaretopics/Consent/Consentgeneralinformation/index.htm

[7] Human Tissue Authority about the HTA http://www.hta.gov.uk/about_hta.cfm

[8] Medical Research Council Policy and Guidance Consent to take placed in research http://www.mrc.ac.uk/PolicyGuidance/EthicsAndGovernance/InformedConsent/index.htm

[9] Knowledge of the laws in consent in surgical trainees. Hamilton P Bismil Q. Ricketts DM. Annals of the Royal College of Surgeons England. 2007;89:86.

GOLDEN RULES OF CONSENT

1.   In an emergency situation a clinician's duty of care to perform a procedure that is in a patient's perceived, or known, best interests supersedes all other things.

2.   Consent is permission giving from a patient to a clinician.

3.   Patients have the right to give permission or withdraw it for their own reasons, at any time.

4.   Adult patients [age 18 and over] are presumed in law to have full decision making capability.

5.   Persons aged under 18 may have capacity, in other words children can make decisions for themselves in certain circumstances.

6.   Autonomous decisions made by patients are valid decisions even if they are against clinical advice i.e. patients can refuse clinical advice.

7.   Consent is about process and system with decision making as opposed to form filling.

8.   Mental Health legislation is about the clinical management of mental diseases or disorders per se and must not be used as a lever to clinically manage an unrelated physical condition i.e. override autonomously given consent.

9.   To make a quality decision requires quality information first.

10.   Decision making requires time.

11.   No adult may give consent on behalf of another adult unless they hold a power of attorney.

12.   If in doubt seek senior advice.

DEFINITIONS

AGE OF MAJORITY

The age of majority in England and Wales changed from age 21 to age 18 on 1ˢᵗ January 1970. In Scotland it is 16. Note there may be some trust deeds drawn up before that date where the age of majority will still be 21. Note that in other countries the age of majority i.e. becoming an adult does vary. On attaining the age of majority the person is classed as an adult with the rights that that society confers upon an adult subject to laws [1].

AUTONOMY

The right or power to govern oneself; self-determination. An autonomous being is one that has the power of self-direction, possessing the ability to act as it decides independent of the will of others and of other internal or external factors [2].

CONSENT

To give permission [3].

CAPACITY

US legal definition; Having legal authority or mental ability. Being of sound mind [4]. It may be taken to mean "having decision making ability".

EMERGENCY

A sudden unforeseen crisis (usually involving danger) that requires immediate action [5].

INVASIVE CLINICAL PROCEDURE

A clinical action with involves the penetration of a tissue, organ or viscus. [Author's definition]

REFERENCES

[1]   HM Revenue and Customs Home page search age of majority http://www.hmrc.gov.uk/manuals/dmgmanual/html/DMG46001/10_0092_DMG47063.htm

[2]   u-s-history.com general interest glossary http://www.google.co.uk/url?sa=X&start=0&oi=define&q=http://www.u-s-history.com/pages/h1451.html&usg=AFQjCNHxjrdCeao3b8OAVcf62KjAvZZZsQ

[3]   The Chambers Dictionary. Chambers Harrap Publishers. Editor. C. Schwarze. 1993. Page 363.

[4]   US government. terms http://www.id.uscourts.gov/terms-cd.htm

x

[5] Google search engine. Define emergency http://www.google.co.uk/search?hl=en&defl=en&q=define:emergency&sa=X&oi=glossary_definition&ct=title

CHAPTER 1

Basic Law and Consent

Abstract: The proof that consent has been given by a patient lies with a clinician as part of their duty of care within the tort of negligence. An adult may give consent for themselves however if they are incapable or a child then another appropriate adult, except in an emergency situation, must be included in the discussion about consent for the patient. There is case law and legal doctrine that underpins such an approach and aspects of statute law that also apply.

INTRODUCTION

This section is about the basics of law pertaining to consent. Readers who wish to elucidate further opinion or text should consult standard legal reference books on the subject.

In the matter of capacity please refer to the chapter **DECISION MAKING ABILITY**.

Concerning consent in clinical practice the emphasis is upon the principle that no person may touch another person without the first person granting permission to do so. An assault has been defined as follows "an assault is committed where the defendant intentionally or recklessly causes the victim to apprehend immediate unlawful personal violence" [1]. That a doctor may fall foul of the law in consent has been reported and so censured by their licensing body the General Medical Council. In 1998 it was reported in Hospital Doctor, a doctors' weekly newspaper [2] that a consultant paediatric cardiologist was suspended for six months after a six year old girl died following a heart operation whereby the procedure was carried out without parental consent.

The burden of proof is upon the clinician that consent was freely given. "if a defendant in court wants to claim they believed the other person was consenting, they will have to show they have reasonable grounds for that belief"- from the sexual offences act 2003 [3].

For a clinician to perform a clinical procedure, except in an emergency life threatening situation without consent, renders the clinician liable for a civil, or possibly criminal, charge of assault. The possibility of a criminal charge results from the removal of crown immunity (see before). This places the first source of evidence upon the clinician in any allegation as they must demonstrate that permission granting was freely given by the person offended.

Other aspects of law pertaining to consent involve Tort which basically is defined from older language as "wrongdoing" i.e. "French word meaning "wrong". Body of law which determines rights and liabilities when property is damaged or a person is injured, through negligent or intentional conduct" [4].

There are effectively 4 elements to Tort in clinical negligence

Element 1	there has to be a duty of care, and
Element 2	there has to be a breach in that duty of care, and
Element 3	there has to be causation i.e. harm due that breach, and
Element 4	there has to be proximity i.e. that the harm due to that breach is logical and proportionate. In other words, if a surgeon operates on the right hand and the left ear falls off that is not proximate to the procedure performed [5].

All four elements must be present to provide evidence of negligence not partial elements. Elements 1, 3 and 4 are relatively easy to determine in that a) a duty of care is part of a professional's life b) no allegation would occur if not harm was noticed and c) the harm is usually obvious. Consent issues appear when one considers the breach in the duty of care. The defence challenge to the breach in duty of care is the so called Bolam Test [Bolam vs. Friern Hospital Management Committee 1957] whereby a doctor is not deemed to have acted negligently if the practice is supported by a body of opinion by similar professions. This was subsequently 'modified' in 1993 in Bolitho vs. City & Hackney Hospital Authority as to introduce a "reasonableness" test i.e. that the defence through that body of opinion had to stand up to logic. Given that is the professional's duty of care to obtain consent appropriately as outlined above, if consent was not deemed to be taken appropriately then the duty of care can be perceived to be breached. This trails back deeper in that if the consent was incomplete due to improper or incomplete information giving (see **CLINICAL INFORMATION**) the consent and then duty of care falls. A recent example of this was Chester vs. Afshar whereby the surgeon failed to inform the claimant of all the risks of the operation including the one that transpired. Whilst the surgeon *per se* did not operate negligently, the process of information giving leading to consent with full knowledge was deemed to be flawed as a full disclosure of the risks involved was not given [6]. (see **CLINICAL INFORMATION** risks). The defence position in such issues is based upon the doctrine of necessity whereby the clinician acts for the patient's best interests. The dichotomy often arises in duty of care disputes around the principle of necessity as perceived vs. a patient's autonomy to make their own decisions (see **BASIC ETHICS**).

To give permission (i.e. consent) requires information giving of a quality appropriate to the patient otherwise a claim of negligence can arise, often hinging upon the breach of duty of care.

THE AGE OF MAJORITY

As mentioned and referenced in **DEFINITIONS** the age of majority varies by country. In particular with young people a clinician may be confronted with a young person who when resident in their own country is given full rights to consent in compliance with local law. However, as a visitor or resident in another country they may not perceive the difference in the age of majority and consequent rights. The age of majority applies to the country the law is enacted rather than to the citizenship of the person giving consent. Although a minor fact, it has the potential for conflict through misunderstanding. Hoyte from the Medical Defence Union writing in 1996 does give clarification to the concept of minors and children [7] he states that the Family Law Reform Act 1969 established that a young person aged 16 – 17 can give consent for medical, surgical or dental treatment although any major or hazardous procedure should involve a consultation with parents unless such permission is refused by the young person. If parents though a legal process have agreed that an invasive clinical procedure is in the best interests of the young person, yet the young person refuses then the parents retain the power of veto over the young person. In simple terms a young person aged 16 or 17 can say 'yes' on their own behalf if the procedure is in their best interests, but cannot say 'no'.

NEXT OF KIN

There is often a misperception by those close to a patient and some clinicians of the right of the next of kin to give consent on behalf of another adult. *(see also **DECISION MAKING ABILITY** and **WHO CAN <u>GIVE</u> CONSENT**)*. Next of kin has been defined as "the person or persons most closely related to an individual by blood, marriage or a legal ruling" [8].This implies those outside such an arrangement or relationships are debarred from the consent process. The basic premise in law is that only an adult can give consent for themselves unless they lack capacity (see also **DECISION MAKING ABILITY - CAPACITY**). This means that no other adult can give consent on behalf of another adult and so the next of kin have no right to donate consent on behalf of another adult unless they have been given that right in law as an "attorney" *(reference to Capacity Acts)*, or the matter is a subject of human tissue donation in death or death (see **POST-MORTEM CONSENT & ORGAN RETENTION / SPECIMEN RETENTION**).

Person with Parental Responsibility

There are occasions when the parent of a child must decide what is in the child's best interests for a clinical situation. The person who holds such responsibility whilst commonly referred to as the parent is best referred to as the person with parental responsibility as it cannot be presumed that the natural parents are married and so have equal rights. From the Children Act 1989 [9].

1. Where a child's father and mother were married to each other at the time of his birth, they shall each have parental responsibility for the child.

2. Where a child's father and mother were **not** married to each other at the time of his birth—

   a. the mother shall have parental responsibility for the child;

   b. the father shall not have parental responsibility for the child, unless he acquires it in accordance with the provisions of this Act.

3. References in this Act to a child whose father and mother were, or (as the case may be) were not, married to each other at the time of his birth must be read with section 1 of the [1987 c. 42.] Family Law Reform Act 1987 (which extends their meaning).

4. The rule of law that a father is the natural guardian of his legitimate child is abolished.

5. More than one person may have parental responsibility for the same child at the same time

However, from 1st December 2003: an unmarried father who registers his name as the father of the child, on the child's birth certificate, will automatically have parental responsibility, but, this is not retrospective. An unmarried father, whose name appears on the child's birth certificate before 1st December 2003, has no automatic right of parental responsibility and can only acquire this right by order of a court.

This latter point has significance as the age of a child has importance *vis a vis* the father who is unmarried and whose name appears on the birth certificate. There will be a diminishing cohort of unmarried birth-certificate-registered fathers who have no parental rights from 2003 to 2019 when the child will attain rights in consent. It is important therefore that those involved with children and young people and faced with an unmarried father whose name is registered on the birth certificate must ascertain if that father has rights or not relevant to the above date and so age of the child.

THE ROLE OF THE COURTS

A court of law is the final arbiter in a case of dispute in consent. In the first circumstance discussion between the clinician and patient and/or carers must take place. If an issue arises that cannot be resolved then it is wise to seek local legal advice from a solicitor or a Trust legal department. Only in a complete lack of negotiation or resolution should a legal case come to court or, in the case of a child if the clinical welfare of the child is of urgent or immediate concern and there is no resolution to be obtained from, or dispute with, the person with parental responsibility.

STATUTE LAW

There are various legal statutes that govern basic law and this will evolve. Examples include:

The Children Act 2004 [10] concerning the welfare and rights of children

The Human Tissue Act 2004 (HTA) [11]

The Mental Capacity Act 2005 (MCA) [12] concerning decision making ability.

The Mental Health Act 2007 (MHA) [13]

Other parts of the United Kingdom have differing statute laws and so it is important to know the geographical area of legal influence that one is practising in. Particular sections of law will be marked within the relevant section.

REFERENCES

[1]   e-law learning http://www.e-lawresources.co.uk/forum/viewtopic.php?f=65&t=244

[2]   Hospital Doctor 26th March 1998

[3]   Home Office.gov.uk, Adults safer from sexual crime. The Sexual Offences Act 2003 http://www.homeoffice.gov.uk/documents/adults-safe-fr-sex-harm-leaflet?view=Binary

[4]   Adler and Giersch personal injury law. Glossary of common legal terms. http://www.adlergiersch.com/legal.cfm#T

[5]   Definition of Torts 1999 by Ronald B. Standler. http://www.rbs2.com/torts.htm

[6]   nes NHS Scotland / courses / northern presentation by Medical Protection Society on consent http://www.nes.scot.nhs.uk/courses/north_presentations/documents/Scottishconsentpresentatio nupdated20.12.05.ppt

[7]   The principles of consent. Hoyte P. International Journal of Orthopaedic Trauma. 1996; 6: 74-77.

[8]   The Chambers Dictionary. Chambers Harrap Publishers. Editor. C. Schwarze. 1993. Page 922

[9]   The London Gazette gov.uk/acts/acts1989 The children Act 1989 (c.41). http://www.opsi.gov.uk/acts/acts1989/ukpga_19890041_en_2

[10]   Office of public sector information.gov.uk/acts/acts2004 the children Act 2004 (c. 31) http://www.opsi.gov.uk/acts/acts2004/20040031.htm

[11]   Office of public sector information.gov.uk/acts/acts2004 http://www.opsi.gov.uk/acts/acts2004/20040030.htm

[12]   Office of public sector information.gov.uk/acts/acts2005 http://www.opsi.gov.uk/acts/acts2005/20050009.htm

[13]   Office of public sector information.gov.uk/acts/acts2007 http://www.opsi.gov.uk/acts/acts2007/20070012.htm

CHAPTER 2

Basic Ethics and Consent

Abstract: There are many ethical principles that guide doctors and underpin their approach to care. In recent times an ascendant principle has been autonomy – the right of a person to make decisions for and about themselves.

INTRODUCTION

This section is about the basics of ethics pertaining to consent. Readers who wish to elucidate further opinion or text should consult standard legal reference books on the subject. Clinical ethics and consent are intimately entwined and there is much written about specifics in standard referenced and textbooks.

Medical, or clinical ethics can be like philosophy in that you can choose which ethical principles you wish to apply. However, there are four established principles: Autonomy, Beneficence, Non-maleficence and Justice [1].

AUTONOMY

This is the strongest of these bioethical principles in relation to consent. In decades past there has been a silent view that the professionals were in charge of clinical things through their unique knowledge and training placing the patient in the subservient position. This amounted to paternalism whereby "doctor or nurse knows best". Within the four principles above the professionals adhered predominantly to beneficence and non-maleficence as their sole guiding principles. Various case law issues and a changing society have resulted in autonomy taking an ascendant position, and even a supreme position above that of beneficence and non-maleficence. Autonomy is about the individual's right to self determine what happens to themselves. This came particularly to the fore with the decanting of mental health patients from institutions into the community. The advocacy that encouraged this was that individuals should be free to make their own decisions albeit with support – the right of self-determination. This also means that an adult who can make a decision of an autonomous nature can only give consent for themselves and no one else. It is their body and their disease and so their decision. No other adult can act on their behalf unless decision making has been lost. Similarly the adult cannot offer the decision to someone else to make on their behalf unless it is a matter of a loss of capacity.

Autonomy can pose difficulties for clinicians if the decision made by the patient is not aligned with the view of the professional. This is outlined in the case of Re C, (1994) which established that a person who has a view that is alternate to that of the professionals is not wrong provided that the decision fits within the principles of capacity. (see **DECISION MAKING ABILITY - CAPACITY**). The decision may be not be logical to a clinician but is valid if the person has capacity (decision making ability) and so is free to exercise this, even if the person has a mental disorder. The issue was outlined in the Law Commission report N⁰ 231 in 1995 on Mental Incapacity *(no longer available unless requested)* in Lord Justice Thorpe's guidance in the landmark case of treatment refusal i.e. Re: C 1994 whereby the elements of decision making were clearly described (see **DECISION MAKING ABILITY - CAPACITY**). Further validation of this can be seen in law from other author's analysis i.e. MacLean "the right of a competent adult to refuse consent to medical treatment is well recognised in English law (*S v McC*; *W v W* [1972] AC 24; *Re T* (adult: refusal of medical treatment) [1992] 4 All ER 649, CA.). It is founded on the right to autonomy and the principle of (respect for) autonomy" [2].

So it apparent that the ethical principle of autonomy is now upheld through case law (1994) and now through statute i.e. the Mental Capacity Act (2005). This shows how strong society through ethics and law supports the right for an individual to make autonomous decisions particularly in the area of consent.

BEST INTERESTS

This relates to both the professional's view of what clinical management is in professional best interests and what the patient views as to be in their best interests. The professional must ensure that their proposed management is in line with what would pass the Bolam Test subject to Bolitho scrutiny; in other words "is the proposed plan of action reasonable on clinical grounds reflecting upon the disease / disorder management and upon the patient i.e. the host of that disease / disorder?" This then must be placed before the professional and the patient. Then the patient on digesting this information must decide what is in their best interests. At this juncture the professional is in the passive role and must not apply duress to the patient who must establish in their own mind what is in their best interests. This process of determining best interests also constitutes part of the decision making process of the patient (see **DECISION MAKING ABILITY - CAPACITY**). It is important to note that under the MCA that the patient's perception of their best interests may not concur or align with those of the profession or professional as established in Re: C. this does not mean that the patient is irrational or suffering as mental disturbance. A person's best interests may be determined by culture, previous personal experience or religion e.g. Jehovah's Witness patients. Provided that the person has capacity to make a decision then that decision is valid for them even if does not align with medical or nursing opinion i.e. the principle of autonomy. Exploring best interests are part of the professional's duty of care and to some degree are responsibilities of the patient. The dreaded "what would you do doctor?" is to be deflected as the patient is the host of the disease and so has an autonomous decision to make against their own best interests of how the disease should be clinically managed. It will take time with tact and patience to assist a reluctant patient to make their own decision. However, should the patient remain adamant that they will not comply with the systems approach to capacity and consent and fall to "whatever you think is best" - such issues must be documented clearly to prevent any future confusion. In other words a record of what transpired at the material time. The documentation must include an assessment of capacity and what the perceived best interests are, or, that have been declared. Best interests are unique to an individual whereas clinical best interests often cover a group of people with the same or similar condition.

REFERENCES

[1] Priory.com. Medicine on-line Medical Ethics Dr Ben Green http://www.priory.com/ethics.htm

[2] Caesarean Sections, Competence and the Illusion of Autonomy Alasdair R Maclean 1999 available from http://webjcli.ncl.ac.uk/1999/issue1/maclean1.html

CHAPTER 3

Decision Making Ability – Capacity

Abstract: Capacity is also known as competence and is about decision making ability. The simplest basis of capacity is the ability to understand and retain information and then to weigh it up and then decide. It is presumed in law that all adults have such ability and it is also taken that older children (who may be referred to "young persons") can have the ability. However, if an adult or child / young person lack such a complete ability then strong measures must be in place to protect them.

INTRODUCTION

Following on from law and ethics is the basic presumption that adults can make autonomous decisions for themselves by themselves. This decision making ability is known as 'Capacity' or 'Competence'.

The Mental Capacity Act 2005 has enshrined the principles of capacity in statute [1].

WHO THE MENTAL CAPACITY ACT AFFECTS

The Act pertains to everyone aged 16 and over and provides a statutory framework to empower and protect people who may not be able to make some decisions for themselves, for example, people with dementia, learning disabilities, mental health problems, stroke or brain injuries [2].Every adult has the right to make his or her own decisions about health, legal, financial and other matters and is assumed to have capacity to do so unless it is proved otherwise [3]. The Capacity Act 2005 is quite specific in its nature and clinicians must familiarise themselves with it through training. Issues such as "best interests" documentation etc are an essential requirement to show compliance with the Act.

The Basics of Capacity

The Law Commission report № 231 Mental Incapacity outlined the case of Re: C and the determinants behind the analysis of decision making. There three elements to be considered viz.

Element 1: an ability to **understand** and **retain** the imparted information.

Element 2: **believing** the information.

Element 3: **weighing up** and **arriving at a choice** i.e. the decision.

With the introduction of the Mental Capacity Act 2005 the second element has fallen out of favour as it is impossible to test "belief" of either party – the giver or the receiver whereas the other two elements are testable, giving a two stage test.

Part of the decision making by the patient will be their assessment of their best interests (see **BASIC ETHICS**).

SIMPLE TESTING OF THE TWO STAGES

To test stage 1 (understand and retain) it is reasonable to ask the person to repeat back to the person imparting information and taking consent what they have understood. This brings into bearing another legal principle of "at the material time". If the information imparter can understand what has been relayed back to them then this supports the fact that the original recipient has understood the information and retained it for that material time.

To test stage 2 (weigh up and decide) then immediately following on is an exploration of the weighing up process hopefully encouraging the person to display their reasoning without comment or duress and then the decision.

This then effectively completes the process of assessing capacity. The difficulty remains if doubt about capacity exists – in which case, as in many things, the advice of someone senior must be sought for those who are less experienced or knowledgeable.

ADULTS

The presumption in law is that those who have attained the age of majority have capacity. As noted previously this may vary by country. The MCA outlines the principles clearly viz.

1. A person must be assumed to have capacity unless it is established that he lacks capacity.

2. A person is not to be treated as unable to make a decision unless all practicable steps to help him to do so have been taken without success.

3. A person is not to be treated as unable to make a decision merely because he makes an unwise decision.

4. An act done, or decision made, under this Act for or on behalf of a person who lacks capacity must be done, or made, in his best interests.

5. Before the act is done, or the decision is made, regard must be had to whether the purpose for which it is needed can be as effectively achieved in a way that is less restrictive of the person's rights and freedom of action."

YOUNG PEOPLE AND CHILDREN

The age of 16 is taken as the age of acquisition of untainted capacity by the MCA. The principles as applied to adults are really no different when engaging with young people or children. A child may indeed be quite able to make decisions the so called, -"Gillick

Competent" child aged 16. This arises from Gillick v WestNorfolk and Wisbech Health Authority [1986] AC 112;- when it was held that, were a child is under 16, but has sufficient understanding in relation to the proposed treatment to give (or withhold) consent, his or her consent (or refusal) should be respected. However, the child should be encouraged to involve parents or other legal guardians.] [4] the process of scrutinising Gillick competency is known as the Fraser Guidelines [5]. Yet, the danger in using such descriptions is to presume it is easy to ascertain the "haves" and the "have-nots" by a simple process. Given that the law underpins adults as having *de facto* consent making ability which does not somehow apply to younger people then it is an obligation to assess the younger person's decision making ability routinely. It is also wise to withdraw from terminology such as "Gillick Competent" as it seemingly invests full power than may actually be fragmentary or partial. It is better to state and document that the young person or child has, or has not, capacity without an appellation such as 'Gillick' or 'Fraser'.

LACK OF CAPACITY

A person lacks capacity if they fail to understand and/or retain and/or believe and/or weigh up and/or decide upon the information that has been imparted. It is important for the giver to assess beforehand the person's ability to decide if there is a reason to do so either through a concomitant medical condition, stress or young age.

The MCA defines such a person who lacks mental capacity as "(1) For the purposes of this Act, a person lacks capacity in relation to a matter if at the material time he is unable to make a decision for himself in relation to the matter because of an impairment of, or a disturbance in the functioning of, the mind or brain. (2) It does not matter whether the impairment or disturbance is permanent or temporary."

Under such circumstances a clinician remains bound by their duty of care and must act for the patient's best interests. This then requires the clinician to determine, rather than presume, what these best interests might be and ensure that they are upheld, even if they do not align with the proposed clinical action.

Potential difficulties may arise in the future with legal cases whereby the temporary nature of a lack of capacity might be challenged at a future date should a risk consequence arise. Clinicians should be aware of the descriptive terms used in the MCA and document decisions fully.

In an adult with a chronic disturbance of the mind or brain such as dementia then the clinician must seek out either an advance decision document (also known previously as an Advance Directive or Living Will) or discover from those closest to the patient what they understand, or not, to be the best interests of the patient and so comply or align the clinical actions accordingly. In the absence of such advice or information then the clinician is bound to act according to clinical needs under a duty of care. Should no person or written decision be made in advance then a clinician can use consent form 4 (see **FORMS OF CONSENT**) to document the process.

In a child who fails capacity then it is the role of the person with parental responsibility, or in their absence or dispute, a solicitor or Trust legal department and ultimately a court of law to decide. The issue at the core is what is in the child's best welfare interests.

In all circumstances whereby the process has snagged it is important that the clinician maintains full documentation in the records and seeks more senior advice as permits or is available.

REFERENCES

[1]   Office of public sector information.gov.uk acts 2005. http://www.opsi.gov.uk/acts/acts2005/ukpga_20050009_en_2

[2]   Department for Constitutional Affairs Home Legal Policy Mental Capacity index http://www.dca.gov.uk/legal-policy/mental-capacity/index.htm

[3]   Department for Constitutional Affairs Home Legal Policy Mental Capacity index mibooklets guide 3 http://www.dca.gov.uk/legal-policy/mental-capacity/mibooklets/guide3.pdf

[4]   Your rights. Org. UK. The Liberty guide to human rights search Gillick http://www.yourrights.org.uk/your-rights/chapters/the-rights-of-children-and-young-people/parental-resposibility/key-area-s-of-parental-responsibility.shtml

[5]   Royal College of Nursing Signpost guide for nurses working with younger people. Sex and relationships education. http://www.rcn.org.uk/__data/assets/pdf_file/0008/78578/002021.pdf

CHAPTER 4

Clinical Information

Abstract: To use capacity wisely requires access to information. Information quality must be full and neutral in content and cover alternatives as well as potential risks. The quality of imparted clinical information must be of the highest standard, relevant and pertinent to the individual patient. Regarding risks, specific attention to frequency based upon sound knowledge can be ascertained by using standard methodologies and principles as used in non-clinical risk management situations. Allowance has to be made for patient perception as well as professional's perception in the arena of quality.

CONSENT EXPRESSIONS

*"Informed consent" is a term that is used frequently in clinical parlance. However, "informed consent" is actually an American legal term. It is not actually defined in UK law despite its frequent usage. "Express" and "valid" consent are also used as adjective descriptors. However, all consent should be express and valid. There is no place for invalid consent or consent that is not expressive. The term "knowledgeable" is defined as "possessing knowledge", and so the term **Knowledgeable Consent** is more appropriate as it implies that the patient has the knowledge donated by the clinician, to make a decision upon, appropriate to the patient's circumstances. Knowledge and capacity equates to validity and not information alone. No information equates to no consent, as there is no information to make a decision upon when a person acts autonomously to ascertain what is in their best interests. Whereas knowledge through information giving of quality and decision making based upon this with time to think constitutes strength in consent giving and receiving.*

INFORMATION VERSUS KNOWLEDGE

Information has two components:

COMMUNICATION STYLE AND FORMAT:

The style must be appropriate to the recipient of the information including appropriate language, level of literacy and understanding. The format may be verbal or written in an appropriate style [1].

The manner of imparting information relates to two components; the giver and the receiver. The giver must assess the ability of the receiver to take on board the information i.e. establish the best forum and format to deliver the information. This may be oral, in writing or a video or pictures, or in combination. It is important that the style does not overwhelm the person receiving the information nor that they should feel under duress by time or to appease the clinician.

CONTENT

Patients do wish to know the content of information given to them. Over 80% [2] of patients want to have detailed information about any complications or adverse effects that might happen, including 75% who wished to know about the risk of death. Concerning when such information of complications or adverse effects should be given, 62% of patients requested that the information should be given at the first consultation and on the day of surgery.

There are seven (7) important headings (principles) to anchor information against viz.

1. the reasons for,

2. the nature of,

3. the benefits of,

4. the risks of,

5. the discomforts of,

6. the alternatives to, and,

7. the consequences of not receiving - the invasive clinical procedure

The reasons for, the benefits, the alternatives to and the consequences of not having the invasive clinical procedure are usually self evident. The nature of the invasive clinical procedure usually requires more information as this is in actuality describes the proposed actions.

The General Medical Council gives advice in their 2008 guidance [3] in specific numbered sections as follows:

7. The exchange of information between doctor and patient is central to good decision-making. How much information you share with patients will vary, depending on their individual circumstances. You should tailor your approach to discussions with patients according to:

a. their needs, wishes and priorities

b. their level of knowledge about, and understanding of, their condition, prognosis and the treatment options

c. the nature of their condition

d. the complexity of the treatment, and

e. the nature and level of risk associated with the investigation or treatment.

8. You should not make assumptions about:

   a.   the information a patient might want or need

   b.   the clinical or other factors a patient might consider significant, or

   c.   a patient's level of knowledge or understanding of what is proposed.

9. You must give patients the information they want or need about:

   a.   b. any uncertainties about the diagnosis or prognosis, including options for further investigations

   b.   options for treating or managing the condition, including the option not to treat

   c.   the purpose of any proposed investigation or treatment and what it will involve

   d.   the potential benefits, risks and burdens, and the likelihood of success, for each option; this should include information, if available, about whether the benefits or risks are affected by which organisation or doctor is chosen to provide care

   e.   whether a proposed investigation or treatment is part of a research programme or is an innovative treatment designed specifically for their benefit

10. You should check whether patients have understood the information they have been given, and whether or not they would like more information before making a decision. You must make it clear that they can change their mind about a decision at any time.

DISCOMFORTS

Discomforts include pain, catheters, intravenous or blood lines, tubes, feeding tubes, drains, dressings, monitors, splints etc. A patient may relatively easily accept the risks of an invasive clinical procedure, but if the discomforts are not explained as well, then when the patient does complain of a discomfort the clinical staff may downplay this aspect of the patient's care. However, the discomfort is personal thing to the patient who may be having their first experience of a procedure. If a described discomfort is ignored or downplayed then a complaint may arise as the patient feels ignored and their genuine concerns to them are being dismissed. It is therefore very important to discuss discomforts; and to remember that risks are not the same thing as discomforts.

RISKS

It is wise to avoid "soft" or seemingly "safe" words such as "complication" or "side effect" which may be an attempt by the clinician to ease the burden of the consequence of the risk. Whilst the clinician may be comfortable with the risk it is the patient who may, or is likely, to suffer the risk and its consequence and so it is personal to them. Within the principle of autonomy what Patient 'A' might easily accept as a risk, Patient 'B' might not accept. This will influence their decision making capacity set against their perception of their best interests. Further, risks differ from discomforts. Substantial or significant, or common / frequent, or other important risks must be imparted to the patient; this may include the risk of death. No matter how uncomfortable a clinician may feel about discussing death it can be an outcome either as a direct result of the disease and its management or the general status of the patient's other health or family history. The conveyed risks are what the patient wants or needs to know, rather than what the clinician thinks the patient may want to know. How a patient perceives a risk and any consequences that may then occur may differ substantially from how the clinician perceives the same risk and so it is always a personal event to the patient. It is impossible to be prescriptive about what risks should be imparted as the judgement of what must or should be imparted is as much a feature of the patient's desire for knowledge as the clinician's ability to know or evidence such risks.

RISK INFORMATION QUALITY

There are various means of communication between a clinician and a patient including oral, written and video systems independently or in collaboration. Quality and style is important both for the giver and the receiver. One question that the author has asked of trainee doctors at a registrar stage or above is the following "is it reasonable to give 10 common risks of any given invasive clinical procedure"? Universally the answer is "yes". The trainees are then asked to list 10 risks with haemorrhage and infection as the first two. It is not uncommon for trainees to struggle to achieve the ten. When the trainees are pushed to grade the severity of the risk their responses improve. However, when asked to then quantify those risks by frequency of occurrence the trainees again have difficulty.

Consider a common clinical invasive procedure – insertion of a chest drain. It is possible to reach 10 risks by including nerve and organ damage including lung and heart damage. However when asked to quantify a risk such as intercostal nerve damage or puncturing a lung then the information is less forthcoming. Often a trainee will give a value such as 1% however when pushed to evidence this value often it is a presumption or a guess or "I think I remember reading it somewhere". There is a paucity of evidence of risks pertaining to the procedure as such, yet, such procedures are commonly performed daily within healthcare without any apparent risk. Within the arena of consent if a patient has to make a decision based upon knowledge then the quality of that knowledge must be good and if the source of the knowledge is uncertain then the decision itself is less than a quality one.

It is also interesting to consider comparing two invasive procedures a) removal of a bunion and b) lumbar puncture. The former procedure may be performed under general anaesthetic whilst the latter under a local anaesthetic. What are the risks of each? Does the person taking consent provide more information for the bunion procedure than the lumbar puncture because the former is under a general anaesthetic? The risks of bunion surgery under general anaesthetic probably are much less than a lumbar puncture which has an intimate relationship to the spinal cord, yet the formality of consent in writing applies more to bunion surgery than lumbar puncture. This seems illogical if the risks of lumbar puncture are greater either in severity or frequency.

The imparting of risk information has been the subject of recent legal deliberations in civil clinical negligence cases. In Chester vs. Ashfar [2004] UKHL 41; [2004] 4 All ER 587 the matter eventually turned not upon harm (causation) that had occurred but imparted information i.e. risks about the procedure. The surgeon had failed to adequately inform the patient and so the risk that transpired (in this case Cauda Equina syndrome from prolapsed disc surgery) was not available for the patient to consider. Further, in this judgement, there was an acceptance that a risk of 1-2% frequency must be declared irrespective of anything else. Even more recently (2008) in Birch vs. University College London Hospital NHS Foundation Trust [England and Wales High Court (Queen's Bench Division) [2008] EWHC 2237] the claimant successfully sued as information about the comparative risks of one form of investigation (angiography) over another (MRI) were not imparted and the patient suffered the known harm from the more invasive procedure i.e angiography – she had a stroke which would not have occurred with the non-invasive MRI. The consequence of legal judgements in such cases suggests that for a significant risk the failure to impart the risk of a frequency of 1-2% may be judged as a failure in a duty of care [4].

FORMS OF RISK

There are two forms of risk. The first is the generic risk of performing an invasive clinical procedure on a person irrespective of any other factor i.e. the risks that are common to that invasive clinical procedure at all times. The second are the risks related to the individual patient and there own risk factors e.g. obesity, cardiovascular disease etc. This can be illustrated by the following example. Consider the invasive clinical procedure of tonsillectomy. There are common risks to this procedure irrespective of upon whom the procedure is performed. Now consider two different patients who warrant the procedure of tonsillectomy. The first is a 30 year old fit, active joiner with no previous medical history or family history of a disease. The second is a 30 year old patient with Down syndrome with congenital heart disease and deafness. The technical procedure and attendant surgical risks of tonsillectomy are common to both patients however there are likely to be further or more significant risks with the Down syndrome patient than the "normal" patient. The conveyance of risk to both patients will differ both in content and format and so bespoke risk communication is essential.

SEVERITY OF A RISK

This is often reasonably easy to convey as the consequences of a pathological event are familiar territory to the clinician. However, this may be of more significance to the patient as for them this may be the first or only time that the procedure will be performed upon them.

Consider the following scenario. A surgeon is required to remove a benign growth from a spinal column near the spinal cord. The pathological consequence of a risk may render the patient partially paralysed. Within the surgeon's mind although this is a tragedy of sorts it is within the province of surgery that risks occur and there is remedial therapy to help or support the patient. However, if the patient is a self employed steeplejack and the sole breadwinner for a family the consequences of paralysis are possibly more severe in sociological terms than the pathological terms if such a risk should occur. The severity of a risk will have a perceptive component within the ethical principle of autonomy.

FREQUENCY OF A RISK

From the above it is within more difficult territory for the clinician to accurately and evidentially convey the frequency of a risk without presuming. Whilst the general severity and frequency of a particular risk may be well known, other moderating factors to that risk are less likely to be well known; such as the effect of the relationship between the host and the disease. Research in generic risks may be patchy or be presumed to be universal ignoring for example the competency of the person performing the procedure. Journal texts do provide risk rates by procedure but this is not a commonality. Medical defence organisations have databases of harm uncovered through the litigation process and the National Patient Safety Agency accrues incidents to its database. Yet such data is not in the common or open source arena and is not analysed to its generic specificity or accuracy as representative by the Royal Colleges or the professionals' associations. The hard evidence of generic risk rates is hard to come by and may be out of date at the time of publication. Further, as outlined below, ensuring the risk rate is relevant and bespoke to the needs of an individual requires a greater knowledge and data analysis of what can be found within the public domain. Without knowledge of a risk rate it is difficult for a patient to assimilate the information pertinent to their own disease and circumstances. Further the professional's view of risk rates may apply to outcomes rather than inherent risks per se. The author conducted a snapshot survey in December 2007 using Google as a search engine. The search string was "laparoscopic sterilisation risk". From the search results, up to 80 results, there were 21 NHS organisations in the public domain that had a positive hit. Of these 21 the information leaflet about the risks of the procedure were assessed. Only 5 of 21 (23%) organisations made any mention of a risk rate for a risk and this was usually confined to a single risk rate for a single risk i.e. "failure of the procedure" without reference to the source, including the official advice from the National Institute for Health and Clinical Excellence. There was neither ranking of risk by severity nor a risk rate for other mentioned risks. There was no mention of any risk rates in the remaining 16 (77%) organisations. Whilst a snap Internet survey is nothing more than illustrative it does suggest that organisations have either no knowledge of risk rates or are failing to publish them. The National Patient Safety Agency does provide incident occurrence [not clinical risk] rates, however these are reported back to senior staff in the individual organisations on a confidential basis.

To elevate risk frequency to more substantial evidence requires a system that allows for this. One possible method other than ongoing audit of procedure outcomes is a modified risk assessment.

USING RISK MANAGEMENT TOOLS TO EVALUATE RISK IN CLINICAL PRACTICE

The standard risk assessment format is the following:

The standard risk assessment model (based on industry) to approaching a problem such as this is as follows: A. IDENTIFICATION: A1 what could go wrong? A2 How could that happen? A3 what would be the effect? B. ANALYSIS: B1 how often is this likely to occur? B2 How severe is the effect if it did occur? B3 what would be the cost if it did occur, - (time, finance, down time etc). C. CONTROL: How do you C1 eliminate the problem, C2 avoid the problem, or C3 make the problem less likely to occur.

By modifying this approach to only evaluate only elements A1, B1 and B2 i.e. what, frequency and severity generically for each invasive clinical procedure would go a long way to improving the quality of evidence of risks attendant to an invasive clinical procedure being preformed.

It can be useful to consider risks to be identified under several headings:

1. Anatomical risk: to adjacent organs and structures

2. Physiological risk: - disturbed function of structures

3. Biochemical risk: - disturbed body parameters

4. Pathological risk: - long term, or distant, effects

5. Psychological risk: - dealing with any consequences.

Whilst surgical invasive clinical procedures would appear to be the most dominant territory this however relates more to attendant factors such as the use of anaesthesia. However, the principles of identifying the risks and quantifying them by severity and frequency apply equally to non-surgical practice such as lumbar puncture, or chest drain insertion, and invasive cardiological, gastro-intestinal, haematological, invasive respiratory and radiological procedures.

It is worth remembering that an established risk of 1:100 is an actual number in that the risk will occur once per hundred rather than might occur at a rate of once per hundred as the evidence has been taken from data accrued and analysed, rather than supposed.

In this way a solid profile of risk information is established that is generic to the procedure and related to the clinician's audited practice. Thereafter it is a matter of customising the information to the specific needs of the patient. Bespoke risk information proportionate to the patient is the quality ideal that ensures that the provenance and architecture of the information is to an established format with an evidence base through audit data collection. Further information from resource evidence such as a Royal College audit can be used to strengthen the audit process of data quality and so risk information. In this way with an underpinning audit process to the modified risk assessment approach the risk information remains dynamic and pertinent both to the clinician, the patient and in a contemporaneous manner. This allows for quality benchmarking and archive of clinical risk information to demonstrate a progress to enhanced quality data and information gathering and usage. At an extreme is also allows for comparisons in practice to further enhance the quality of information used.

It can be difficult to convey a risk rate to a patient in a meaningful way that converts a mathematical certainty to a descriptive term. Some meaningful work has been done [5]. This table reviewed the risk of an individual dying in any one year or developing an adverse event. The term 'high' was used for a risk estimate of greater than 1:100, 'moderate' for a risk estimate between 1:100 and 1:1000, 'low' for a risk estimate of between 1:1000 and 1:10 000, 'very low' for a risk estimate of between 1:10 000 and 1:100 000, minimal for a risk estimate of between 1:100 000 and 1:1 000 000 and 'negligible' for a risk estimate less than 1:1 000 000. The perspective of a 'minimal' risk to a clinician may be 1:100 yet research suggests that such a term is reserved for risks less than one in a million and a 1% or greater risk should be taken as high. Using this information can create a decision making grid about whether to inform a patient or not of a risk. By aligning risk frequency against risk severity it is possible to generate a decision making grid. Such a grid can involve both professional and lay input and help arrive at a commonality of agreement i.e. a form of Bolam Test in advance. Such as grid and process has been described before [6]. An example is shown in the table below:

Table 1: severity vs. frequency grid for a single identified risk

		RISK SEVERITY		
		SEVERE	MODERATE	LOW
RISK FREQUENCY	HIGH > 1%			
	MODERATE 0.1% - 1%			
	LOW 0.01% - 0.1%			

In this option the cells coloured in grey represent a collaborative viewpoint of what is not required to be told to a patient or written on a patient information leaflet. This is a point of agreement. The unfilled cells represent severity – frequency values which it is agreed that it will be mandatory to convey to the patient should the patient so choose. In this way a collaborative team approach of professionals and lay people can make a decision based upon evidence fact which itself creates a nodal decision making point of what it is reasonable to communicate or not. This approach, although more difficult to formulate is likely better than either pole of "do not tell the patient anything in case the patient becomes distressed" or "tell the patient everything we will give them the lot". The example above is not an absolute and will likely vary for each risk with differing decision about frequency vs. severity being conveyed. The system does allow for professional decisions to be based upon reason and collaboration and be retained for future reference within a dispute. It would be prudent to document within a formal committee or group structure through minutes the rationale that supports the common decision.

Other perceptions of risk rates and their communication to patients can differ though. Gigerenzer and Edwards [7] suggest ways of communication or expression that translates medical statistical risk jargon into more meaningful information for patients to comprehend. They suggest that the facts do not need to be distorted, but rather that they be taken from the lexicon of the statistical or medical environment and be placed within the comfort zone of a patient's comprehension and ability to understand. Paling [8] points to visual aids as necessary and using information and not just data to illustrate communication and information perception.

The concept of judging whether a risk rate is applicable remains in dispute. In 1997 Sir Magdi Yacoub an eminent international transplant surgeon (Poynter v Hillingdon Health Authority [1997] 37 BMLR 192) as defendant was cleared of negligence in an area concerning disclosure of risk. The Independent newspaper "Yacoub cleared of negligence" Jeremy Laurence Health editor Thursday 24th April 1009 page 3 declared that Sir Maurice Drake (judge presiding) ruled that the parents of a child who suffered brain damage after a cardiac arrest after a heart transplant had been properly warned of the risks. Further in the piece *"Sir Magdi told the court the risk was so small – less than 1 per cent – that he would not tell parents about unless specifically asked. Transplant surgeons yesterday agreed it was impractical, and could be unwise, to tell patients of every conceivable risk. Bob Johnson, a kidney surgeon and chairman of the British Transplant Society said: "we tell patients about the classical risks – of dying, of the organ being rejected, of side effects of immuno-suppressant drugs. But you can't go through every remote risk" "* It is interesting that Calman *q.v.* a year earlier had used the term "high" to describe the risk of dying from any cause at 1% or greater yet in transplant surgery a risk of 1% or less this was described in court as "small". A decade later on this imbalance of what is high risk or not at 1% remains undecided. Yet again 1:100 from research i.e. 1% means that the risk has occurred once in every hundred times. For an individual to make a determination for themselves in what may a single event in their lives does ask the question of whether disclosure should be more complete, if clinicians actually have the evidential answers to risk rates.

Others have attempted to transmute numerical values into meaningful expression. Earlam *et al* [9] compared their work with others and evaluated percentages as "Certain" for 100%, "Almost always" for 95%, "usually" for 70%, "fifty-fifty" for 50%, "sometimes" for 20% "almost never" for 5% and "never" for 0%. However, given that many risks fall into the 5% or less category and 5% from established evidence equates to an actual occurrence of 5 in 100 occasions of factual occurrence their lexicon tends towards the unlikely occurrence of a risk. Further, a "certain" occurrence of 100% is no longer a "risk" but a definite eventuality as part of the procedure. Finally for a surgeon to have an evidenced occurrence of 5 in 100 times may appear small to the surgeon when imparting risk values, but for 5 of the patients the event actually occurred which in their terms is 100%. Perhaps one should be wary of attempting to find the common ground of communication between clinician and patient and seek to ask the patient how they would like the risk to be imparted, after all it is the patient who will bear that risk and it is an individual decision based upon the patient's beliefs and understanding i.e. autonomy and capacity.

ENGAGING WITH THE PATIENT

In 2001 an editorial in the British Medical Journal reflected upon the engagement of patients when medical decisions are made [10]. The authors acknowledged that many decisions in healthcare are complicated and require time for the decision to be made. They also comment that in a study of breast cancer management 34% of women wanted to delegate responsibility for clinical management to their doctor. Such a value (over one third) if extrapolated to consent suggests that the rigours of decision making which underpins consent may be too much for the patient to bear. The communication of risks should be in the form of a dialogue in simple and relevant terms reflecting the patient's needs rather than the clinician's presumption of what is important [11]. For a clinician to act as a guide or partner, like a mountain guide who does not carry the burden but shows the client how to achieve what they want within a context of safety and ability, they must understand the difficulties in communicating risks and the style and format [12]. Whilst there has been an acknowledgement that risk information is important in medical decision making it has taken until 2003 for such matters to rise up the doctors' flagpole of awareness [13, 14].

INFORMATION AVAILABILITY AND QUALITY

The development of the World Wide Web has made access to information much better. Ellamushi *et al* [15] browsed the Internet in 2001 for information on 5 neurosurgical terms. The information quality was assessed by a clinician. The information quality was graded from 4 (full information) to 1 (irrelevant Website) via grade 3 (partial information) and grade 2 (information not useful). There was a wide variation in quality per procedure at best 52% of sites achieved grade 4 quality for one condition down to 3.5% for another condition. This latter condition scored 70% for grade 2 and grade 1 combined. Further, several sites displayed broken links or were dead-to-access. Whilst there is an abundance of information on the world-wide-web it is apparent the actual availability and quality varies greatly. There is no standard gatekeeper of information on the world-wide-web, and in particular clinical information about certain conditions and their clinical management. This means that a patient who accesses the Internet for information has no knowledge of the quality or provenance of the information, nor is it bespoke for their purposes. If a patient enters a consultation pre-informed from the Internet with the illusion of knowledge then there is an inherent danger in that what transpire thereafter may be a fraught consultation and a distortion of the flow of information that leads to proper and duress-free consent giving.

PATIENT'S PERCEPTIONS

In 2002 Langdon *et al* examined the effect of a written patient information sheet [16] and found that there was a statistical benefit for information being imparted in writing and that imparted orally, but that recall of information was better in the written information group. Further patients preferred written information even though in this procedure the risk of fatality was discussed. Whilst a further study [17] was concerned about issues around the hospital admission rather than consent it was shown that the patient has a desire for information particularly for females but not by age. In 2006 Akkad *et al* [18] noted that 10% of the study group (women) did not know what they had agreed to although 82% were aware that there were risks with surgery. The patient perception was that almost 50% thought that the form was there to protect the hospital from litigation and almost two thirds thought that the consent form gave the doctor control over what happened. The authors conclude that there is a disparity between "consent theory" in the biomedical model and what happens in real life.

INTER-PROFESSIONAL ASPECTS

Browning in 1997 [19] showed disagreement and limited concordance between a patient's perspective and that of a surgeon's analysis for symptoms. However, further on as to whether surgeons agree it was shown that for a set of criteria there was a wide range of opinion. This part of the study was within a peer group! Perhaps more worryingly Houghton *et al* [20] concluded that 37% of junior doctors taking consent had little understanding of the procedures only a decade ago. McManus and Wheatley commented in 2003 study [21] that many surgeons (56%) did not provide written information despite General Medical Council issued guidance with wide variation in the amount or type of risk information imparted including page 80 "One surgeon claimed to never mention any of the given complications". Hoyte from the Medical Defence Union writing in 1996 page 75 does give clarification to the concept of junior staff [22] he states that "Ideally, therefore, consent should be obtained by the consultant for the case".

From the literature above it would seem that the expectations or understanding of consent may be better within the patient arena than the professionals' arena despite significant advice and direction from established peer groups and authorities.

Evaluating and imparting risk information between professionals and between professionals and patients remains a difficult area of communication. The underlying mathematical evidence for specific risk occurrence is poor generally and per procedure and so this means that the imparting of such information is also poor. Further, there is increasing evidence that clinicians are not certain in what format and to what degree risk information i.e. knowledge should be imparted. Whilst it is wise to base such communication to an individual level, the research tends to seek a commonality for groups which obfuscates the concept of individual autonomy and capacity. It appears that indeed currently "one man's meat is another man's poison" in the matter of consent and risk imparting from the view of either party – the transmitter and the receiver.

REFERENCES

[1] Parliamentary and Health Services ombudsman . Home. Publications. Consent in cardiac surgery. Good practice guide. http://www.ombudsman.org.uk/improving_services/best_practice/cardiac05/consent.html#relaying

[2] Patients' views on consent for surgery: a questionnaire survey. Chandrsenan J. Morris MWJ. Williams JL. Annals of the Royal College of Surgeons England *(supplement)* 2007; 89: 140-142

[3] General Medical Council. guidance. ethical guidance. consent guidance. sharing information. http://www.gmc-uk.org/guidance/ethical_guidance/consent_guidance/sharing_information_and_discussing_treatment_options.asp

[4] Clinicians must share risk information properly with patients. McILwain J.C. Health Care Risk Report. 2008.vol 15 issue 2. Page 12-13

[5] On the state of Public Health Calman KC. Health Trends vol.28 No.3, 1996 Table 1.2 page 84

[6] Clinical Risk Management: principles of consent and patient information. McILwain JC. Clinical Otolaryngology. 1999, 24, 255- 261 Table **1**

[7] Simple tools for understanding risks: from innumeracy to insight. Gigerenzer G. Edwards A. BMJ, Sep 2003; 327: 741– 744.

[8] Strategies to help patients understand risk. Paling J. BMJ, Sep 2003; 327: 745– 748.

[9] Obtaining consent for an operation: a choice of words or numerical probabilities? Earlam R, Rizwan-Hasib M, Tross S, Morrris G. Clinical Risk 2007; 13: 45 - 52

[10] Engaging patients in medical decision making. Kravitz RL. Melnikow J. BMJ, Sep 2001; 323: 584 – 585.

[11] Communicating Risks. Edwards A. BMJ, Sep 2003; 327: 691– 692.

[12] Patients Understanding of risk. Thornton H. BMJ, Sep 2003; 327: 693– 694.

[13] Influence of the law on risk and informed consent. Mazur DJ. BMJ, Sep 2003; 327: 731– 734.

[14] Commentary: informed consent and risk communication in France. Moumjid N. Callu MF. Commentary: communicating risk in the United Kingdom. Powers M. BMJ, Sep 2003; 327: 735– 736.

[15] Is current information available useful for patients and their families? Ellamushi H. Ganesalingam N. Kitchen ND. Annals of the Royal College of Surgeons England. 2001. 83. 292-294.

[16] Informed consent for total hip arthroplasty: does a written patient information sheet improve recall by patients? Langdon IJ. Hardin R. Learmouth ID. Annals of the Royal College of Surgeons England. 2002; 84: 404-408.

[17]   What Patients really want to know about their surgery. Mehta S. Powell L. Cooper JC. Annals of the Royal College of Surgeons England (supplement) 2003; 85: 360 - 363

[18]   Patients' perceptions of written consent: questionnaire study. Akkad A. Jackson C. Kenton S. Dixon-Woods M. Taub N. Habbiba M. BMJ. 2006; 333:528-9.

[19]   Do patients and surgeons agree?: The Gordon Smyth Memorial Lecture. Browning GG. Clinical Otolaryngology. 1997; 22: 485-496

[20]   Informed consent: patients' and junior doctors' perceptions of the consent procedure. Houghton DJ. Williams S. Bennett JD. Back G. Jones AS. Clinical otolaryngology. 1997.;22:515-518

[21]   Consent and complications: risk disclosure varies widely between individual surgeons. McManus PL. Wheatley KE. Annals of the Royal College of Surgeons England. 2003;85: 79-82.

[22]   The principles of consent. Hoyte P. International Journal of Orthopaedic Trauma. 1996; 6: 74-77.

CHAPTER 5

Types of Consent

Abstract: The degree of recording of consent is generally proportionate to the potential risks that may occur or significance of the procedure. There is the usage of standardised consent forms for various purposes. The duration of consent does remain elusive as to exact guidance.

IMPLIED, VERBAL AND WRITTEN CONSENT

It is unreasonable to consider completing a written form every time consent is taken. Whilst consent imparting, giving and taking is a process that is dynamic a written form is purely a document at a time and a place concerning what has been written down. Such a form rarely encompasses the totality of the process. Nevertheless there are many occasions when consent is accepted by the actions of the patient. The following applies to invasive clinical procedures.

IMPLIED CONSENT

This can be taken to exist after information has been given to the patient or, that they are familiar with the procedure, the action of the patient is logical and appropriate for the procedure being performed. A good example is venepuncture whereby when asked for permission to give a blood sample the patient holds out their arm for the procedure. There is an implication that the patient knows what is going to occur and why. It would be unreasonable to expect a consent form to be completed for such a procedure given that any risks or discomforts are of limited or no consequence. In simple terms implied consent is valid for simple procedures which take place whilst the patient is alert, seated and not in distress. Further, it rarely necessary to impart a complete amount of information as one would do for a formal more significant procedure with consequences. Non-invasive clinical procedures may also fall into this area.

VERBAL CONSENT

This is a granting of authority to the clinician by the patient in a verbal manner. The imparting of information to the patient may be also given orally or by written text. Such a process is usually reserved for intermediate invasive clinical procedure in which the patient is alert, the procedure is elective and local or no anaesthetic agent is to be used. Examples of this include lumbar puncture, chest drain insertion, catheterisation, radiological interventions of a minor nature. It would be acceptable custom and practice that verbal consent is taken for procedures that do not render the person in any way incapable of exercising their capacity to withdraw consent during the procedure for any reason. However, the more the significant the procedure or the more common or significant the risks then the greater the likelihood the clinician may elect to have written consent in a standardised form. Whatever the clinician elects for, verbal or written, any verbal consent must be clearly documented. The choice to use a formal consent form or not is that of the clinician. In simple terms an invasive clinical procedure performed at the bedside with or without local anaesthetic and of a low consequence of risk may be achieved with verbal consent. Non-invasive clinical procedures may also fall into this area.

WRITTEN CONSENT

This is a more traditional and better understood system within healthcare delivery. There has however in the past been a belief that written consent equates to a *"Carte Blanche"* to do whatever the clinician deems fit or necessary. This is not the case. A consent form is purely an agreed format of recording information and authority exchange at a specific date. Further, consent forms imply that the giving of an anaesthetic agent is part of the process, but consent giving for anaesthesia *per se* is not a standard practice. A recent journal debate remained in favour of anaesthesia being retained as an integral part of the consent process and form within the UK [1,2,3]. Yet Lloyd *et al* in 2003 [4] noted that (surgical) SHOs (Senior House Officers) were more likely to warn of anaesthetic risks 40% than SpR's (registrars) at 33% than consultants at 24%. The process of written consent is by its very nature more laborious and time consuming yet it may be the sole evidence that a clinician has that proper information and authority exchange occurred. The completion of the form is discussed below and in **WHO CAN TAKE CONSENT.**

CONSENT FORMS

For general purposes a written form is used when the patient will enter the environs of an operating theatre and will have a general or significant anaesthetic that may render them to be without capacity. However, the Department of Health Form 3 also covers circumstances whereby an invasive clinical procedure may be performed outside an operating theatre and without a general anaesthetic. In such circumstances Form 3 may be used whereby previous verbal consent was expected. In its essence Form 3 is mainly for minor invasive clinical procedures previously relating to the concept of minor surgery with or without local or small regional anaesthesia.

CONSENT FORMS IN COMMON USE

There are four forms introduced and approved by the Department of Health from April 2002. All Department of Health forms have clear instructions to clinicians about consent and how to use of each form. It has been an obligation for all NHS bodies in England and Wales to adopt and use these forms. The purpose is to achieve commonality of documentation across the NHS. Further advice is available from the Department of Health [5].

FORM 1: Patient agreement, usually an adult, but a competent young person may sign, and involves the use of General Anaesthesia. This is the main form that has been commonly understood to be in use particularly in surgery and hospital practice. However, modern medical interventions may also require the use of general anaesthesia as a supplement to performing a procedure that is not the traditional surgical manner. In other words the concept of the form refers to a) adults and b) general anaesthesia but is not exclusive to surgical procedures.

FORM 2: Parent and/or child's agreement. This form is reserved for a parent or person with parental responsibility (see before) to use; with either person able to countersign and involves the use of General Anaesthesia. This form parallels form 1 but is aimed directly at children / young people and those who have parental responsibility.

FORM 3: Patient / Parent agreement but when General Anaesthesia will **NOT** be used, but regional or local anaesthesia will be used. As outlined above this covers those situations whereby no general anaesthesia is used yet the invasive clinical procedure has a significance either from consequential risk severity or frequency yet is more than one would expect from a simple annotation of an agreement made verbally. There is no prescriptive list of what procedures are or are not inclusive for use with this form, it remains a professional's own decision. It is logical though to consider a written record made to a formal manner for procedures that attract a significant or common risk such as lumbar puncture, chest drain insertion, suprapubic catheterisation, and other such invasive clinical procedures that are common clinical procedures performed outside the traditional operating theatre environment. Further, clinicians who perform "minor" surgery either within a hospital or general practice environment may consider the use of such a form. From the perspective of say a skin cyst i.e. the disease entity, if the cyst appears within a hospital referral environment then its host [the patient] is likely to be subject to a formal process and system of evaluation and form filling around consent. If the cyst appears within a general practitioner's environment and is to be removed there may not be such formal approaches to either consent or its record given the special and more intimate relationship between the general practitioner's patient and more limited size of practice. In other words the general practitioner will likely know the patient better than when the patient enters a more corporate environment of a hospital setting. The decision to use form 3 or not is not proscribed and so it is to each individual practitioner to decide upon its use, unless an organisation sets down rules and procedures to follow such as in exclusion list of procedures.

FORM 4: the patient lacks capacity. In these circumstances clinical staff will determine what the patient's best interests are both clinical, social and spiritual etc. such solicitation will necessarily involve those close to the patient which may or may not include partners, next of kin, or carers; in other words those who know the patient best. Next of kin or relatives have no automatic right to either be first consulted or to make the determination. The determination of best interests is made by the clinical team after consultation. There is no necessity for two consultants to sign this form. The core issue is the determination of best interests both clinical and non-clinical, and the recording of how determined and how assessed.

Forms 1-3 have a section that allows a patient to apply a restriction such as "I do not wish my ovaries to be removed" in a proposed hysterectomy, or, "I forbid blood products to be placed in my body" for Jehovah's Witness patients. There is also a space for advance decision statements and withdrawal of consent. Risks and any potential procedures of necessity must also be documented along with type of anaesthesia and use of an interpreter.

Form 4 has areas for completion as statements that include details of proposed treatment, assessment of capacity, assessment of best interests, and involvement of those "nearest and dearest" and their affirmation as well as space for a second opinion. However, there is nothing officially written that states that a second opinion is mandatory; even if it is taken to be a prudent option by a clinical professional. The concept that "two signatures are required" is neither an actual requirement nor obligation unless the treatment is complex or there is disagreement between the clinicians and those "nearest and dearest".

OTHER CONSENT FORMS

Within an organisation there may be a need for bespoke departmental consent forms. Such forms may include those for Medical Photography, Research, Audit, foetal remains and non-invasive clinical procedures whereby consent in writing is deemed appropriate. There is no standard guidance on such forms as to format and content and each organisation must direct itself as to the quality and usage of such forms.

DURATION AND REAFFIRMATION

Consent has no specified longevity. It could be argued that when consent is taken and it has a relevance to a material time then it exists in perpetuity. However, whilst such a concept may give comfort and ease of administrative management to an organisation or an individual it presumes that a patient's mind is set in stone with no opportunity to re-think or amend their views as their own life experiences and thoughts prevail. There is however no specified time limit on consent although Hoyte from the Medical Defence Union writing in 1996 does give clarification to the concept [6] by suggesting that "A couple of months is probably an acceptable interval, although this issue has not been tested by the courts".

To circumvent this issue of duration and the potential need to rewrite a new consent form which might invoke a different person being involved the Department of Health consent forms invoke the principle of reaffirmation. In other words the process begins at the initial signing of the form for an elective procedure. When the patient is admitted for the definitive procedure then the section:

Confirmation of Consent (to be completed by a health professional when the patient is admitted for the procedure, if the patient has signed the form in advance)

On behalf of the team treating the patient, I have confirmed with the patient that s/he has no further questions and wishes the procedure to go ahead.

Signed   Date

Name (PRINT)   Job title

The purpose of this is to "reactivate" i.e. continue on the consent process, or, to reaffirm or modify as need be the form. Should there be a material difference between what was proposed originally and what is available or proposed on admission then a new consent form should be completed to ensure that the issues are not cluttered. The old form must not be destroyed but an annotation made upon it that it is superseded and a note made in the clinical record as to the reasons why an amendment requiring a new form has been made. This may seem over bureaucratic however it is the "living" form that declares the patients wishes and so transference of authority through consent. It is an important section and should not be undertaken in a trivial manner.

THE NEW NHS FORMS IN ACTION

Ibrahim *et al* in 2004 analysed the new consent forms at a pre-assessment clinic [7].Two hundred patients were examined with 100 in an 'old form' group and 100 in a 'new form' group. The new form scored better in relation to the information source (doctor or nurse) and the name of any complication particularly infection, thromboembolism, haemorrhage and death. The use of the Internet as a resource was 5% for the new form and 3% for the old suggesting a reliance on personal imparted information. Probert in 2007 looked at the new consent form in relation to fractured neck of femur [8]. Their work showed surprising and some disturbing aspects of form usage 5 years after the new consent form was introduced. The study group was 175 case records of which 32 (18%) still had an old form and 6 (3%) had no consent form. Whilst major risks were noted discomforts (pain, stiffness) were also listed as risks. Noteworthy as well that in patients who lacked capacity the authors refer to the use of form 4 as "consultant consent" although this is not actually specified in the Form 4 guidance. It is wise that senior doctors reflect upon consent and capacity given the situation, but consultant input is not actually mandatory. They comment that (in 2007) it is the junior staff who often take consent. They suggest separate consent forms i.e. procedure specific forms to harmonise and standardise risk information being imparted. This is an ideal however as some inherent issues such as the large archive required, the differences between individual consultants per procedure *(see above)* and the physical need to print out the consent forms in A3 size. The rationale behind A3 size folded forms is to eliminate the risk of documents falling apart in time and to avoid sharp staples. There are precious few A3 printers connected to computers in many organisations. Further, standardised forms belie the ability to customise a form to a patient's specific needs. Written patient information sheets can be standardised to the model of 7 topics previously suggested along individual surgeon's thoughts. Thereafter a signed copy of this information sheet can be filed as evidence with the completion of the following box on the information sheet at the end of the sheet,

BOX 1. Completion of information sheet for filing

IF FILING <u>THIS</u> COPY OF THIS INFORMATION SHEET IN THE CASE RECORD

NAME OF CLINICIAN <u>GIVING</u> INFORMATION:

YOUR SIGNATURE: DATE   /   /

NAME OF PERSON <u>RECEIVING</u> INFORMATION:

THEIR SIGNATURE: DATE   /   /

This allows standardised information to be given in writing to the patient and filed as a true copy for evidence with flexibility on the standard consent form for bespoke risk information that a patient may need.

NON-INVASIVE PROCEDURES AND CONSENT

The standard consent forms apply to those procedures that use anaesthesia or not, and are invasive. However, there are therapies or treatments that use procedures that are regarded as non-invasive in the conventional way such as radiotherapy, oral chemotherapy. It is often taken to be the case that such procedures or therapies are taken on implied consent in that the primary consulting clinician has agreed with the patient about a modality of treatment that is non-invasive. The secondary clinician inherits the consent by implication similarly to an anaesthetist accepting consent for anaesthesia from the surgical team and patient. Whilst many of the undesirable effects of such procedures are discomforts, risks can and do occur. Consider radiotherapy for a head and neck cancer; the discomforts of radiotherapy include reddening of the skin, dry throat and a loss of saliva whilst the risks include a breakdown of tissues and a fistula or a failure to cure. Similarly in HIV therapy the effects of medication can include discomfort such as diarrhoea but also risks of elevated blood lipids and possible cardiovascular effects. Whilst a procedure in itself mat be noxious to the tissue and body, similarly radiation and ingested therapeutic chemicals may carry discomforts and risks which may bas a great or greater than for an invasive clinical procedure. By addressing such issues along the headings previously discussed in **PATIENT INFORMATION** then it is reasonable to propose consent to proceed from the patient to the clinician for the execution of non-invasive procedures which may make use of Form 3 or an alternative developed by an organisation. This then harmonises the principle of consent to other clinical territories. A semi-parallel concept occurs in psychiatry with the use of a contractual arrangement between the clinician and the client to ensure an adherence to a proposed treatment plan to enable compliance. Such a contractual level of agreement is unnecessary yet some mode of acknowledging consent given the gravitas of the therapy / procedure makes logical sense.

REFERENCES

[1]   Formal Consent in Anaesthesia. McILwain J.C. Health Care Risk Report. 2007.vol 13 issue 8. Page 15

[2]   How anaesthetists deal with consent. Bogod D. Health Care Risk Report. 2007.vol 13 issue 8. Page 16

[3]   Consent for anaesthesia – a legal overview. Volpe H. Slingo C. Health Care Risk Report. 2007.vol 13 issue 8. Page 17

[4]   The new consent form: are we performing informed consent? Lloyd T. Millett A. Garcea *et al.* Annals of the Royal College of Surgeons (supplement) 2003;85:354-355

[5]   Department of Health. Policy and Guidance. Health topics. Consent. Consent key documents. Consent   form. http://www.dh.gov.uk/en/Policyandguidance/Healthandsocialcaretopics/Consent/Consentgener alinformation/DH_4015950

[6]   The principles of consent. Hoyte P. International Journal of Orthopaedic Trauma. 1996; 6: 74-77.

[7]   The new consent form: is it any better? Ibrahim T. Ong SM. Saint Clair Taylor GJ. Annals of the Royal College of Surgeons England. 2004;86:206-209

[8]   Surgery for fractured neck of femur – are patients adequately consented? Probert N. Malik AA. Lovell ME. Annals of the Royal College of Surgeons 2007;89:66-69.

CHAPTER 6

Consent - When and Where

Abstract: In general the proximity to information giving is to when, and so where, consent taking should occur provided that duress is not applied.

EMERGENCY SITUATIONS

The form is secondary to a true emergency. The time and place for any form completion should be when the patient is most settled and less distressed yet retains clarity of mind that has not been amended by chemicals or significant pain or distress due to an intervention. The MCA notes that any disturbance of the brain or mind even on a temporary basis may render the patient to be without capacity. However, this must be balanced against a clinician's duty of care to act promptly within the patient's best interests to save life.

ELECTIVE PROCEDURES

The definitive consultation is the wisest time to begin or take consent. At this juncture the information relevant to the clinical decision will be available e.g. investigation results. At this point the clinician is at their most informed and so able to convey their opinion easily to the patient. The requirement that has been traditional on the completion of the consultation is to ask "do you want to go on the waiting list?" and then encourage the form to be signed as a completion of the administration and as likely as not to psychologically affirm the patient's commitment to go ahead. Yet, this process may not help as the patient may feel rushed to conform to "the system". It would be reasonable to suggest that when the consultation is complete and an agreed verbal decision made by both parties that the form is then proffered to the patient. The patient can then complete the form then and so enter the waiting list at this point, or, take it away to contemplate it. Thereafter in the latter case when the patient returns the form, the waiting list position can be activated. The patient may feel that this disadvantages them, however, if 25% – 50% do likewise then the waiting list actually shortens and accommodates those who have made a decision in their own time related to their own circumstances.

PRE-OPERATIVE ASSESSMENT CLINICS

There are neither actual rules nor guidance about who can operate such clinics or when they should occur. There is logic on the listing consultation that includes consent taking that a primary pre-operative screening occurs to optimise any medical deficiencies that may exist prior to surgery rather than waiting to a short period before surgery and then adjusting the clinical status to suit operative and anaesthetic necessity. The usual per-operative system employs a visit to the hospital one week or 2 weeks prior to surgery and anaesthesia. Often a screening system is in place utilising trained nursing staff using a pro forma and algorithm of assessing basic clinical necessity. This can be supplemented for the specific proposed procedure using a competent and trained nurse or a doctor from within the speciality familiar with the proposed procedure.

Consent affirmation at this juncture is to rekindle the consent process to make it more contemporaneous and to ensure no changes to any attendant issues have occurred in regard to the procedure, nor that the patient has changed their mind or needs further information. If done well at the initial consultation this process should be smooth. However, circumstances may change and the consent form may need to be rewritten, in which case the same rules as before apply. Again it is wise to document within the case record any significant amendments or new forms.

Any advance decisions or changes in capacity may also need to be addressed particularly in those people who have made an advance decision or changed an old one and for those who may have appeared to lose capacity in the interim wait.

CHAPTER 7

Who can <u>take</u> Consent?

Abstract: As times change so has the role and nature of the person taking consent. No longer is it a case of simply signing a form. The information giving to the patient relies upon a person who is knowledgeable about the procedure and can answer questions. There is no legal demarcation zone between doctors and others concerning who can take consent and it is also proportionate to whether the consent taker is taking consent for procedures that they will perform themselves, or, are taking consent on behalf of another – delegated consent taking. There are indeed official statements about delegating consent.

BASIC REQUIREMENTS

The standard view is that the person who is to perform the procedure should take consent. However, this is not always possible on logistical grounds as the operator may not be available at the time of surgery, or, that it is accepted practice that consent taking can be delegated. In the latter case (see below) it has to be accepted that the delegate is acting for the most senior person who was involved in the decision making consultation. To impart information and then receive consent is usually a continuum involving the one person i.e. the giver and receiver is the same person. In this way the patient can be assured that there is no disarticulation in the process. When a person imparts information using the previously described format of;

"1. the reasons for, 2. the nature of, 3. the benefits of, 4. the risks of, 5. the discomforts of, 6. the alternatives to, and, 7. the consequences of not receiving the invasive clinical procedure"

It implies that there is an understanding and knowledge of the procedure. The ideal concept of an ability to be competent to perform the procedure as well as communicate it is fraught with logistical problems given the modern methods of economic healthcare delivery. Competency to perform a procedure has within it an implication of understanding and knowledge, yet, for a patient making a decision all that is actually required is a person with the knowledge and communication skills to respond to any query; such a person may not actually be technically competent to perform the procedure, or is in training, or is a delegate competent to perform the task.

DOCTORS

Traditionally doctors have had the sole province of procedure management and so are taken to be invested with knowledge and experience. For many invasive clinical procedures this is the case and in many procedures and those which are more significant or complex doctors are the best repository of knowledge and so ability to convey information. Yet, as seen before (see **CONSENT FORMS**) the task of consent taking may befall those most junior for logistical or other reasons and yet these are the people with least experience and so least knowledge.

Doctors are often and are usually capable of imparting consent information, yet this task is being increasingly shared or delegated to other clinical health professionals.

NURSES AND MIDWIVES

Readers should take the term 'nurses' used hereafter as incorporating nurses and midwives.

With the development of nurses to more senior clinical positions and speciality skills the task of delegating and informing consent to nurses is advancing within NHS organisations. Further, senior nurses now function as autonomous practitioners performing procedures that were previously only within the clinical province of doctors and training doctors in procedures traditionally the role of doctor-trainers. For their autonomous practice nurses can and usually do take their own consent for those procedures. Further though as they develop progressively they are trained in, and assimilate, knowledge of invasive clinical procedures that doctors perform. In these circumstances nurses can be ideally placed to be information givers and consent receivers as they remain within post for longer periods than doctors who rotate their jobs on a cyclical basis of between 4 and 6 months duration, or, may be attached to a single consultant trainer. Other permanently employed senior doctors such as Staff Grade doctors or Associate Specialists can also fulfil this role but this depends more on their contractual commitments. Junior staff including nurses should never participate in information giving – consent receiving without supervision and training and should never have such tasks displaced to them for convenience.

OTHER HEALTHCARE WORKERS

In general other healthcare workers will take consent for procedures that they autonomously perform and are trained in e.g. phlebotomists and venepuncture.

DELEGATION

Delegating Consent

Essentially this requires a transfer of authority in such a way that both the healthcare professional and the patient are protected. For a doctor to delegate consent to a more junior doctor there is given advice from the doctors' licensing body – the General Medical Council (GMC) and the British Medical Association (BMA) as well as the Senate of Surgery of Great Britain and Ireland.

OFFICIAL VIEWS ON CONSENT AND DELEGATION

The Senate of Surgery of Great Britain and Ireland ,

"The surgeon's duty of care" 1997. "Surgeons should inform competent adult patients aged 16 and above of the nature of their condition, along with type, purpose, prognosis, common side effects and significant risks.........." [1]

General Medical Council

GMC; Consent: patients and doctors making decisions together. 2008 [2]

> Para 26 : "if you are the doctor, undertaking an investigation or providing treatment, it is your responsibility to discuss it with the patient. If this is not practicable you make sure that the person you delegate to is suitably trained and qualified, has sufficient knowledge of the proposed investigation or treatment, and understands the risks involved, understands, and agrees to act in accordance with the guidance of the [GMC] booklet."

> Para 27: If you delegate, you are still responsible for making sure that the patient has been given enough time to make an informed decision, and has given their consent, before you start any investigation or treatment.

GMC; Consent: patients and doctors making decisions together. 2008 [2].

However this advice is subject to a different view. PMETB notes that doctors in training can only take consent for procedures that they a\re deemed competent to perform *(see **Doctors in training** section below)*. However, this advice has been modified in September 2009 to align with GMC guidance in that both trainee and supervisor must agree that the trainee understands the intervention and its attendant risks; rather than being able to perform competently.

BMA Consent tool kit 2007 [3]

 "The BMA considers that the **doctor** who **recommends** that the patient should undergo the intervention **should have responsibilit**y for providing an **explanation** to the patient and **obtaining** his or her **consent**. In a **hospital** setting this will normally be the **senior clinician**. In **exceptional circumstances** the **task of reaffirming consent** can be **delegated to a docto**r who is suitably trained and qualified, is sufficiently familiar with the procedure and possesses the appropriate communication skills."

(author's emphasis)

This is a different position from the GMC guidance whereby any delegation can be to "a person" and not just a doctor. Further, the BMA reference in delegation is about reaffirmation and not delegation *per se*. As stated the BMA has no view on delegating consent to another health professional.

The emphasis is important. The doctor taking consent must have a comprehensive knowledge of the procedure. The GMC makes it very clear as well that the responsibility of delegation by a doctor to another person must be in circumstances that are not practicable and that person who is acting on behalf of the doctor must have training and knowledge. The GMC holds a doctor's licence to practice.

The Department of Health in its model policy [4] states the following:

1. The health professional carrying out the procedure is ultimately responsible for ensuring that the patient is genuinely consenting to what is being done: it is they who will be held responsible in law if this is challenged later.

2. Where oral or non-verbal consent is being sought at the point the procedure will be carried out, this will naturally be done by the health professional responsible. However, team work is a crucial part of the way the NHS operates, and where written consent is being sought it may be appropriate for other members of the team to participate in the process of seeking consent. Recognising the role of other healthcare professionals in the consenting process.

Department of Health Policy and guidance section 9 [5] states that "The clinician providing the treatment or investigation is responsible for ensuring that the patient has given valid consent before treatment begins, although the consultant responsible for the patient's care will remain ultimately responsible for the quality of medical care provided. The GMC guidance states that the task of seeking consent may be delegated to another health professional, as long as that professional is suitably trained and qualified. In particular, they must have sufficient knowledge of the proposed investigation or treatment, and understand the risks involved, in order to be able to provide any information the patient may require. Inappropriate delegation (for example where the clinician seeking consent has inadequate knowledge of the procedure) may mean that the "consent" obtained is not valid. Clinicians are responsible for knowing the limits of their own competence and should seek the advice of appropriate colleagues when necessary."

Using the GMC guidance as a basis within the Department of Health advice places the majority verdict of a Government Department and the doctors' licensing body as that a doctor can delegate consent taking to another person (fellow health professional) who may not be a doctor provided that certain criteria are met.

DOCTORS IN TRAINING

In 2008 the Postgraduate Education and Training Board [PMETB] issued mandatory notes [6]. In the matter of consent for trainee doctors under Patient Safety 1.4 "Trainees must be expected to obtain consent only for procedures which they are competent to perform". This means that consent could not be delegated to a doctor in training unless they are competent to perform that procedure.

However in September 2009 PMETB changed their mind and now state [7] "1.4 Before seeking consent both trainee and supervisor must be satisfied that the trainee understands the proposed intervention and its risks, and is prepared to answer associated questions the patient may ask. If they are unable to do so they should have access to a supervisor with the required knowledge. Trainees must act in accordance with GMC guidance Consent: patients and doctors making decisions together (2008)." This means that rather than applying a competence test of procedure skills both trainer and trainee must satisfy themselves to the standard of knowledge about an intervention. This aligns with other standard practices in delegated consent.

A SUGGESTED PROCESS FOR FORMAL TRANSFERENCE OF AUTHORITY FOR DELEGATION

The following is the suggested process and system permitting the safe transference of authority from a doctor to a nurse to allow a nurse to act as a delegate for the doctor in consent taking:

1. The nurse must have evidence of skills and knowledge of the proposed invasive clinical procedure(s),

2. The nurse has appropriate approval from their licence holding body,

3. The nurse has formal approval from a supervisory medically qualified consultant, and

4. The nurse is subject to regular audit of the procedure(s). *(This was in the original Department of health advice that is no longer available).*

REFERENCES

[1]   The Royal College of Surgeons England Home Publications and Images Publications Surgeon's Duty of Care - Guidance for Surgeons on Ethical and Legal Issues. http://www.rcseng.ac.uk/rcseng/content/publications/docs/publication.2005-09-15.7076792767

[2]   GMC Home. Guidance for doctors. List of ethical guidance. GMC; Consent: patients and doctors making decisions together. 2008 http://www.gmc-uk.org/guidance/ethical_guidance/consent_guidance/responsibility_for_seeking_a_patients_consent.asp

[3]   BMA. Home. Professional issues and ethics. Consent and capacity. Consent toolkit 3rd edition. http://www.bma.org.uk/ap.nsf/AttachmentsByTitle/PDFconsenttk3/$FILE/ConsentToolKit.pdf

[4]   Department of Health. Policy and guidance. Consent key documents. Guidance for clinicians. Download model consent policy in rich text format. http://www.dh.gov.uk/en/Policyandguidance/Healthandsocialcaretopics/Consent/Consentgeneralinformation/index.htm

[5]   Department of Health. Policy and guidance. Consent key documents. Guidance for clinicians. Reference guide to consent for examination or treatment.

http://www.dh.gov.uk/en/Publicationsandstatistics/Publications/PublicationsPolicyAndGuidan
ce/DH_4006757

[6]   PMETB. Home. PMETB standards and requirements. Generic standards for training.
        http://www.pmetb.org.uk/fileadmin/user/Standards_Requirements/PMETB_Gst_July2008_Fin
        al.pdf

[7]   PMETB. Home. PMETB standards and requirements. Generic standards for training.
        http://www.pmetb.org.uk/fileadmin/user/Standards_Requirements/PMETB_Gst_Sept2009.pdf

CHAPTER 8

Miscellaneous Issues Concerning Communication

Abstract: Not every patient has the same primary language as that of the consent taker and allowances must be built in to any system to allow for this. Equally there has to be an understanding and process that deals with patients who refuse to give consent even if that procedure is in that patient's best interests. The more common usage of "Living Wills" requires some knowledge of their validity and limitations.

COMMUNICATION DIFFICULTY AND PATIENTS

To obtain consent from a patient who is presumed to have capacity requires a transfer of information to allow for decision making. This requires communication skills on the part of the person delivering the information either in verbal or written format. It is an ideal that an organisation will have a knowledge of its local demographics and population to be able to serve the needs of that population either from a language or disability perspective such as poor vision or hearing. This may also require the availability of interpreter services. Failure to support those with disabilities could be an offence under the Disability Discrimination Act 1995, and may prevent consent from being gained. Support for communicating with patients having specific disabilities can be obtained from a range of agencies e.g. Equality and Human Rights Commission [1].

LEARNING DISABILITY PATIENTS

The expression *"Does he take sugar?"* refers to the manner of a clinician speaking to a carer and not to the patient with learning disability directly. A person with learning disabilities has exactly that – difficulty in learning or disabled learning skills. This does not mean that the patient lacks capacity or ability to communicate. They may be unable to relate to standard formats of communication and rely upon others close by or near to them to act as an "interpreter" or facilitator. Full advice is given from the Department of Health in 2001which is an overall explanation of consent and capacity the vignettes are illustrative [2]. The prime issue for the clinician is not to presume that the person with learning disability cannot understand nor decide. It is a matter of communication format not ability.

FOREIGN LANGUAGE

The flow of patients across the world through immigration or tourism occurring more frequently this means that populations are becoming more mixed in language and culture. An insular view of "when in Rome do as the Romans" is no longer tenable if a clinician wishes to make effective communication with patients and seek their consent. Whilst in geographical areas adjacent to airports and sea ports may attract a transient population large cities also attract foreign speaking people who form communities, often speaking in their native language. Such community citizens will eventually abut with the healthcare providers. Given the complexity and breadth of the issue around consent it is important that organisations are aligned with their communities and needs including communication about such needs between professionals and between professionals in other organisations [3]. Information about the consent forms is currently (2007) available as a download in Bengali, Chinese, Greek, Gujarati, Polish, Punjabi, Turkish, Urdu and Vietnamese. The four Department of Health style consent forms are downloadable in Albanian, Arabic, Bengali, Chinese, Farsi, French, Greek, Gujarati, Kurdish Soran, Polish, Pushto, Somali, Turkish, Urdu and Vietnamese.

To facilitate communication a patient with no natural language of English may bring a family member to interpret for them. There is an inherent risk in this. The family member may be indigenous to the UK as a British citizen and be bilingual having a strong ethnic tie to the community with their native tongue in which case the clinician can be reasonably assured that any communication is of a veritable nature. However, if the primary language of the "interpreter" is greater than the other language they use the clinician may feel less than confident that full interpretation has taken place. The clinician then is in the position of the patient effectively – they cannot be fully assured that correct information and the nuances have been transferred. Under such circumstances the clinician may wish to involve a professional interpreter albeit with an added cost. It is not unusual however within a modern setting of UK healthcare delivery that a clinical colleague is available to translate for the clinician which may be the better remedy. Failing all else it is a duty of the clinician to ensure that correct information has been imparted to allow for decision making, by whatever means.

PHYSICAL LIMITATIONS

Those who are disadvantaged by a hearing or visual impairment should also have their limitations realised which may involve utilising other methods of communication.

CULTURAL ISSUES

In certain cultures the patient being a woman may have some limitations placed upon their role as an autonomous patient. This may mean that a husband is present and may "speak for the patient" and "decide" for the patient. There may also be a limitation on consent in regard to "touch" for the purposes of a clinical examination, or, the need to have a chaperone present which also invokes consent for this purpose. Such issues pertaining to actual consent or decision making must be taken into account.

There may be issues of consent pertaining to touching a dead body. In certain religious faiths a person who is not of that faith is deemed "unclean" and if they actually touch that body they transfer their 'uncleanness' to the dead body. In such circumstances there is no presumed consent to touch that body and in such circumstances a member of that religious faith should be consulted. This also extends to organ donation and autopsy.

Further, in single parent families the parent may be at work and a grandparent may be present with a child patient. Whilst it usual and common to proceed to exam the child with the grandparent present however, if consent is to be taken at this consultation then it may not be the case that the grandparent has actual parental responsibility to give consent for the child. The parent can furnish the grandparent with a token of acting *"in loco parentis"* so that the grandparent is acting directly and overtly on behalf of the parent, however this should be established. If the grandparent has no such authority then this needs to be made explicit in a reasoned way and consideration given to another consultation with the single parent present.

REFUSAL

Refusal to give consent may pertain to a person lacking capacity or that the medical viewpoint of the proposed clinical management does not agree with their own personal philosophy, culture, religion or belief.

Issues of refusal by a patient often reflect the issues pertaining to ethics and capacity. A clinician will usually know from their knowledge and competence what is clinically in the best interests of the patient. A clinician is now duty bound to determine what a patient's best interests are to ensure a bespoke clinical programme of management is ascertained and that can be delivered. However, patients are not professionals and in the arena of surgery a patient may have an operation only once in their lifetime whereas the clinician may be performing the same procedure several times per day. Further a patient may give consent at the initial or definitive consultation but thereafter change their mind. Such a change in consent can be frustrating for the clinician and the economical and operational / administrative procedures of that clinician's organisation. If the planned procedure is cancelled due to a change in mind by the withdrawal of consent then the 'procedure slot time' is lost which may not be able to be taken up by another patient. However, patients have a right to change their minds. This effect of changing one's mind and the consequences thereof to the management of a procedures list can be avoided by the quality of the consultation process and information imparting that requires a decision to be made concerning consent.

Further a patient has a right to amend or restrict what is performed within the concept of an invasive clinical procedure. A patient may consent to a hysterectomy but refuse an oopherectomy and state this and declare it in writing on the consent form. A clinician is duty bound to abide by these wishes and so cannot remove the ovaries no matter what the clinical reasoning that would seemingly justify it – even to the perceived level of a Bolam Test. A patient with capacity holds the rights and so the authority to determine what will not be done to their body.

However neither a patient nor a court can force a clinician to perform an invasive clinical procedure if the clinician does not believe that it is in the clinical best interests of the patient. The landmark case was Burke vs GMC which was a matter of future provision of artificial nutrition and hydration and GMC guidance. Whilst the court case was about the GMC advice from this case and its appeal the following issue arose that confirms that a doctor cannot be compelled to provide a procedure if the doctor cannot justify this to themselves on clinical grounds. In other words whilst a patient has the right to refuse recommended medical treatment based upon clinical best interests equally the patient does not have the right to force a doctor to provide a procedure that is against clinical best interests. It is worth setting out the relevant judgement section in its entirety as follows from the court of appeal in 2005 [4]:

50.   The GMC is concerned that these passages suggest that a doctor is obliged, if the patient so requires, to provide treatment to a patient, or to procure another doctor to provide such treatment, even though the doctor believes that the treatment is not clinically indicated. No such general proposition should be deduced from Munby J's judgment, nor do we believe that he intended to advance any such general proposition. So far as the general position is concerned, we would endorse the following simple propositions advanced by the GMC:

i)   The doctor, exercising his professional clinical judgment, decides what treatment options are clinically indicated (i.e. will provide overall clinical benefit) for his patient.

ii)   He then offers those treatment options to the patient in the course of which he explains to him/her the risks, benefits, side effects, etc involved in each of the treatment options.

iii) The patient then decides whether he wishes to accept any of those treatment options and, if so, which one. In the vast majority of cases he will, of course, decide which treatment option he considers to be in his best interests and, in doing so, he will or may take into account other, non clinical, factors. However, he can, if he wishes, decide to accept (or refuse) the treatment option on the basis of reasons which are irrational or for no reasons at all.

iv)   If he chooses one of the treatment options offered to him, the doctor will then proceed to provide it.

v)   If, however, he refuses all of the treatment options offered to him and instead informs the doctor that he wants a form of treatment which the doctor has not offered him, the doctor will, no doubt, discuss that form of treatment with him (assuming that it is a form of treatment known to him) but if the doctor concludes that this treatment is not clinically indicated he is not required (i.e. he is under no legal obligation) to provide it to the patient although he should offer to arrange a second opinion.

It is interesting to think that in social ethics the UK has moved from Medical Paternalism to Patient Autonomy. If the GMC had not won their appeal which overthrew the original judgement in Mr Burke's favour then in a short period of time social medical ethics would have made a polar change from Medical Paternalism to Patient Autonomy to Patient Paternalism.

ADVANCE STATEMENTS

The development of patient determination of their own best interests and declaring them in writing has been evolving over recent decades. The Terence Higgins Trust was an early proponent of placing the future wishes of patients dying of advanced HIV infection into a written format. Other organisations followed suit despite no legal judgement having been handed down form the courts. This pressure resulted in terminology such as "Living Will" and "Advance Directive". Yet, the medical profession had embraced the concept of refusal in the future through a respect for the beliefs of Jehovah's Witness patients. The Jehovah's Witness faith has a particular belief that no blood products should be placed within their body. The Jehovah's Witness faith developed a consent form for that specific purpose of instructing medical and clinical staff to never perform blood administration even should death become the outcome. In 2007 there is a media record of a Jehovah's Witness who refused blood and bled to death [5]. In this case a 22 year old mother died after childbirth having made an express statement that she did not want to have any blood even should she die, based upon her belief. This response to a belief is recognition of capacity and autonomy working together to create a best interests concept in the face of a differing medical opinion of best interests. It is common practice for clinicians when faced with a Jehovah's Witness patient to go and seek a "Jehovah's Witness Consent Form", yet there is clear provision within the current Department of Health consent form to make a declaration along the following lines "I expressly forbid the placement of blood products within my body" or "I expressly forbid the placement of blood products within the body of my child". However, with young people and children it is important that the clinician believes that the child or young person is adherent to that faith and belief and not appeasing the wishes of their parents' belief, in other words the child or young person can make a choice through their own capacity.

However the ethical principle has been in place for some time that a patient who has capacity can make a refusal of medical treatment in the future. However certain conditions must be met viz.

1.   the patient must have made an advance statement in writing.

2.   this statement must be signed by the patient and the signature witnessed after the signature has been made.

3.   the statement must be dated.

4.   the conditions to be met must be exclusive conditions and not inclusive conditions.

5.   the conditions must be clear and unambiguous, yet equally, (for the patient) should not be too precise. A patient who refuses electroshock treatment to restart a stopped heart does not exclude resuscitation *per se* nor cardiac resuscitation by another means such as a chemical like intracardiac adrenaline.

6.   the conditions that must be fulfilled must therefore arise.

7.   the patient must have lost capacity in order to invoke the advance decision.

8.   there should not be a long period between the original decision and the circumstances. Whilst there is no actual rule in this matter as consent degrades with time so does a refusal although taking into consideration that this is a matter of capacity it would be reasonable to suggest that any advance statement is reviewed by the patient every two to three years as both their circumstances, disease and medical advances change.

In 2007 this concept is now on a legal footing in England and Wales with the advent of the Mental Capacity Act. Scotland superseded the rest of the UK in this matter with The Adults with Incapacity (Scotland) Act 2000 [6]. Within this legislation the preferred term used is "Advance Decision" rather than "Living Will" or "Advance Directive". If a person lacks capacity, under this legislation then a person with a power of attorney, Lasting Power of Attorney (LPA) may give or refuse consent for treatment [page 6 - 11.(7).(c)] or continuation [page10. 17. (1) (d)] or the giving of tissue samples [page 77 15 (4)].and is supported by the court [page 14 23. (2) (b)]. However, the Act states that a court appointed deputy "may not refuse consent to the carrying out or continuation of life sustaining treatment" [page 12. 20. (5)] Whilst the current Mental Health Act is in place pending renewal the MCA doe not authorise anyone to give consent for treatment for a mental health condition if they are regulated by part 4 of the current Mental Health Act [page 17. 28 (1) (b)]. Research consent is constrained as well by the MCA [page 17. 30 (1) (a & b) 30 (2) (a & b) - see also 31 (1) & (4) 32 (1) (b) 33 (1) 34 (1) (a & b)].

REFERENCES

[1]   Equality and Human Rights Commission www.drc-gb.org .

[2]   Department of Health. Publications and statistics. Publications. Publications Policy and Guidance. Seeking consent: working with people with learning disabilities. Download. http://www.dh.gov.uk/dr_consum_dh/idcplg?IdcService=GET_FILE&dID=3330&Rendition=Web

[3]   Department of Health. Policy and Guidance. Health topics. Consent. Consent key documents. Consent forms. Downloads. Consent form translations. http://www.dh.gov.uk/en/Policyandguidance/Healthandsocialcaretopics/Consent/Consentgeneralinformation/DH_4001986

[4]   Bailii.org. Databases. England and Wales Court of Appeal (Civil Division) Decisions. [2005] EWCA Civ 1003, [2005] 3 WLR 1132 http://www.bailii.org/ew/cases/EWCA/Civ/2005/1003.html

[5]   On line Newspaper. Guardian Unlimited. Special Report. Medicine and Health. Jehovah's Witness mother dies after refusing blood transfusion. Fred Attewill Monday November 5, 2007. http://www.guardian.co.uk/medicine/story/0,,2205580,00.html.

[6]   The   Mental   Capacity   Act   2005   (MCA)   Office   of   public   sector   information.gov.uk/acts/acts2005 http://www.opsi.gov.uk/acts/acts2005/20050009.htm

CHAPTER 9

Research Consent

Abstract: Following the Second World War, and uncovered atrocities, the Nuremburg Code for medical research was established. This then became the Declaration of Helsinki in 1964 which has eight specific topics detailing consent in research. It is important that any clinician engaging in medical research has access to and adheres to these international guidance topics.

INTRODUCTION

Medical research, or clinical research, has in the past been besmirched with enforced medical experimentation without consent that reached a critical period when the atrocities performed by doctors came to light during and after the Second World War. Experiments to assist doctors to evaluate physiological harm were performed upon unwilling and captive people. As a consequence the Nuremburg Code was drawn up for medical research which has several principles viz.

1. voluntary consent by the participant is essential (autonomy).

2. the expected results should benefit society (utilitarianism).

3. animal experimentation must precede human experimentation.

4. there should be no suffering (non-maleficence).

5. the degree of risk should not exceed expected benefit.

6. protection against death or disability must be built in (non-maleficence).

7. the experimenter or the subject can terminate the experiment at any time.

Trials of War Criminals before the Nuremberg Military Tribunals under Control Council Law No. 10, Vol. 2, pp. 181-182 1949. cited [1] in

National Institute of Health, Office of Human Subjects Research, Regulations and Ethical Guidelines.

The Nuremburg Code of 1949 has been the foundation stone upon which all subsequent medical research has been based and is adhered to. There are many textbooks, university departments and journals devoted to medical research. Within the NHS every organisation will have a formal committee that examines and ratifies medical or clinical research programmes to a formal code of conduct set down from organisations such as the Medical

Research Council. A person wishing to undertake research must have consent from the participant. The Nuremburg Code has been underpinned by the Declaration of Helsinki which began in 1964 and has been taken up by the World Health Organisation and has reached the fifth stage of revision in 2000. There are 32 articles and readers should address the topics directly [2,3]. Of the 32 articles that make up the Declaration of Helsinki articles 8, 15, 22, 23, 24, 25, 26 and 32 directly mention consent giving and taking [4].

The 7 principles of patient information that are pertinent to established procedures apply equally to clinical research viz.

the reasons for, the nature of, the benefits of, the risks of, the discomforts of, the alternatives to, and, the consequences of not receiving the invasive clinical procedure. However, in a newly established or emerging filed of procedure performance some of these principles are less robust that those from established practice. This can make the communication of information more difficult. Whilst the "reasons for" "nature of" "the discomforts" and "the alternatives" are usually self-evident there is less foundation for declaring what is in effect the unknown i.e. the benefits (yet to be established) the risks (yet to be established) and "consequences of not having" (yet to be established). The risks may be supposed yet remain unquantifiable as occurred in 2006 when several young men had a severe reaction to a drug on clinical trial [5].

Whilst there may be many reasons why this event occurred, the effects for the people involved were critical and perhaps unforeseen. The interim report from the Medicines and Healthcare products Regulatory Agency (MHRA) (a government agency) suggested "The MHRA therefore concludes that an unpredicted biological action of the drug in humans is the most likely cause of the adverse reactions in the trial participants" [6]. It is difficult therefore to know how the unknown may be conveyed to a person giving consent within a research setting if the risks are yet to be identified or quantified. The person giving consent must display an act of faith and trust in the research group as new information is being established rather than established knowledge being imparted. This is the reason why clinical research appears bureaucratic, it as much to protect the patient as the future benefits to all.

Consent with knowledge is an underpinning premise of research and readers should direct themselves to their own organisation's Research Committee for guidance, advice and assistance in the matter of design and the inclusion of research and the position of consent.

An authoritative review of research consent and value from 1996 – 2004 for further reading is given by Flory and Emanuel [7].It would be impossible within a book of the panorama of principles to commence a discussion or debate without drowning out the messages of consent appropriate to other issues. Further, given the formality of consent taking for research recognised throughout the modern world and the formal process and system required it is important than any potential experimenter seeks appropriate and formal advice form the appropriate organisational committee.

As a point of note many research committees also supervise audit yet it is important to distinguish between research and audit. Whilst research is an attempt to define what a best practice is or could be, audit is to ensure current practice is being delivered to the levels demanded of research or investigation or inspection.

There are nationally agreed consent forms and these can be accessed for Research Ethics Committee use at the National Patient Safety Agency web site [8] NRES guidance on information sheets and consent forms, page 31 – 34 sections 2.3 & 2.4 for form and Annex B, pages 51 -71 for advice.

RESEARCH CAVEAT: PHARMACEUTICAL CLINICAL TRIALS

In 2004 The Medicines for Human Use (Clinical Trials) Regulations 2004 came into force by Statutory Instrument 2004 No. 1031 and updated to Statutory Instrument 2006 Nº 2984 to comply with Directive 2001/20/EC. This makes provision for Legal Representatives (an "advocate") to consent on behalf of incapacitated adults in respect of participation in therapeutic licensed clinical trials involving pharmaceutical agents i.e. "requires that an incapacitated adult cannot be included in a clinical trial of a medicine without the consent of his legal representative." [9]

Further "Regulation 2 amends Schedule 1 to creates an exception to the general rule that an incapacitated adults cannot be included in a clinical trial unless the conditions in paragraphs 1 to 5 of Part 5 of Schedule 1 have been met; in particular that the adult's legal representative (as defined) has given informed consent. The exception applies only when the following conditions are met: (i) treatment is required urgently; (ii) the nature of the trial also requires urgent action; (iii) it is not reasonably practicable to meet the conditions in paragraphs 1 to 5 of Part 5 (obtaining consent etc); and (iv) an ethics committee has given approval to the procedure under which the action is taken". Note that this statutory instrument applies to clinical trials and not research. It further appears that the Mental Capacity Act applies to research and not pharmaceutical clinical trials. The difference between a clinical trial and research needs to be defined, as the matter of an incapacitated adult and consent-to-participate, may vary according to which definition, circumstance and law prevails.

A clinical trial is an arm of research that tests out a hypothesis, however, in the matter of pharmaceutical agents under The Medicines for Human Use (Clinical Trials) Regulations 2004 it appears that a person with legal powers acting as a Legal Representative can enter an incapacitated person into a pharmaceutical clinical trial without the consent of the incapacitated person. Within the original regulation the definition of a clinical trial is given as follows: "clinical trial" means any investigation in human subjects, other than a non-interventional trial, intended— (a) to discover or verify the clinical, pharmacological or other pharmacodynamic effects of one or more medicinal products, (b) to identify any adverse reactions to one or more such products, or (c) to study absorption, distribution, metabolism and excretion of one or more such products, with the object of ascertaining the safety or efficacy of those products".

A legal representative means [2004 original regulation] not the person involved in the trial and is suitable to so act for these purposes of consent and can give consent for a minor (age over 16). Further, a legal representative who gives consent on behalf of an incapacitated adult in a clinical trial is doing so under the premise of a presumed will to do so by the incapacitated person. Yet who can actually be a legal representative or not, to represent the patient is not clearly detailed and so is not actually defined within the Regulation. Nor is their clear guidance who can, and who cannot be a legal representative in a search of the Medicine and Healthcare products Regulatory Agency.

A Statutory Instrument is a form of secondary legislation or delegated legislation that are usually not actively considered in Parliament and simply just become law. Consultation may occur in the process though [10].

The implications for researchers in pharmaceutical clinical trials involving patients who lack capacity are potentially fraught if no legal representative has been previously determined by the person who has become incapacitated for such purposes. There will be a necessity for any organisation performing such research to ensure that a properly appointed legal representative is created with sufficient authority and knowledge to act in such a role to give consent on behalf of the incapacitated.

Any person seeking to perform medical research in the UK must consult their local Research Ethics Committee. No consent *(inter alia)* = no research.

REFERENCES

[1]   National Institute of Health, Office of Human Subjects Research, Regulations and Ethical Guidelines. http://ohsr.od.nih.gov/guidelines/nuremberg.html

[2]   2.Bulletin of the World Health Organization | August 2008, 86 (8) http://www.who.int/bulletin/volumes/86/8/08-050955.pdf

[3]   World Health Organization, Search: Declaration of Helsinki http://www.who.int/en/

[4]   World Health Organisation. Declaration of Helsinki. Ethical Principles for Medical Research Involving Human Subjects. Bulletin of the World Health Organization, 2001, 79 (4) 373-4. http://whqlibdoc.who.int/bulletin/2001/issue4/79(4)declaration.pdf

[5]   Further lessons from the TGN1412 tragedy. Goodyear MDE. BMJ. 2006;333:270-271 http://www.bmj.com/cgi/content/full/333/7562/270

[6]   Further lessons from the TGN1412 tragedy. Goodyear MDE. BMJ. 2006;333:270-271 http://www.bmj.com/cgi/content/full/333/7562/270

[7]   Interventions to Improve Research Participants' Understanding in Informed Consent for Research A Systematic Review. Flory J. Emanuel E. JAMA.2004;292:1593-1601. http://jama.ama-assn.org/cgi/content/abstract/292/13/1593

[8]   National Patient Safety Agency, National Research Ethics Service, Guidance for applicants http://www.nres.npsa.nhs.uk/applicants/guidance/,

[9]   Office of Public Sector Information. Home. Search. The Medicines for Human Use (Clinical Trials) Regulations 2004 Original regulation in 2004 http://www.opsi.gov.uk/si/si2004/uksi_20041031_en.pdf updated regulation in 2006 http://www.opsi.gov.uk/si/si2006/uksi_20062984_en.pdf

[10]   UK Parliament. www.parliament.uk Home Page. A –Z index. Statutory Instruments. http://www.parliament.uk/documents/upload/L07.pdf)

CHAPTER 10

Consent in Death

Abstract: If an autopsy is required, the role of the Coroner or Medical Examiner has certain legally determined functions. Further, the person who would normally be the consent giver is now dead and so it must be clear whom has the authority and responsibility for the dead including a refusal of autopsy.

INTRODUCTION

When a person dies they are effectively no longer a person and so lose their rights as they become a body not a person. Notwithstanding this there are issues pertaining to death that have to do with dignity and so consent has some role to play in deciding upon issues in the clinical area.

Matters pertaining to death have begun to enter mainstream clinical ethics practice, and in particular right to death. The issues are topical and are currently dynamic with the introduction of the Mental Capacity Act and advance choices and the case of Burke vs. GMC *q.v.* those with an interest in such things should follow the development of both the ethics and law in these matters as they remain dynamic and in flux and so no specific final arbitration can be started for a text.

ROLE OF THE CORONER AND CONSENT

The duty of a Coroner is to enquire into all Sudden, Unexpected, Unexplained, Unnatural, Suspicious or Traumatic deaths. Not all deaths that occur within a district/area are reported to the Coroner. When a death is reported to the Coroner, from whatever source, he/she has a duty to establish certain facts and to be able to do that he has sole control over that deceased person. If the death is reportable to the Coroner and there is a question of Tissue/Organ donation, only the Coroner can give Authorisation to retrieve said Tissue/Organs. Under the Coroners Rules, when the coroner is investigating a death, the coroner has a duty to establish the aforementioned facts. Until the coroner is satisfied as to those facts the coroner has sole control over the body. Once the coroner has established that a person has died from Natural Causes, the coroner will release control back to a family to have a funeral. In Inquest cases, where the death is either unnatural or unexplained only the coroner can release a body after the Inquest procedure has been opened. In Inquest cases which are deemed suspicious, there may be occasions when, even though an Inquest has been opened, there is an ongoing Police investigation, and this may prevent the release of the body until a later date. In other words consent on dealing with the dead person in a Coroner's case rests with the coroner alone.

POST MORTEM: NOT A CORONER'S CASE - CONSENT

Who owns a body after death? No person actually "owns" a corpse, in common law the concept holds that a person may "lawfully be in possession of the body". The difference between ownership and possession is a fine legal one. *(Think note: I can have my friend's pen in my possession but I do not actually own it)*. This person who "lawfully is in possession of the body" will usually be the executor, or the next of kin. In the case of a person who dies in hospital, the hospital management will normally be in possession of the body until the executor or next of kin takes over possession *(see below)*. The legal precedent has been re-enforced "The disposal of the deceased must be left to the claimant as the person currently in lawful possession of the body"

The "next of kin" concept is a relationship to the deceased through "blood and / or marriage". However, the Human Tissue Act 2004 has created a hierarchy of relationships in the matter of "claimant possession". Paragraph 53 on page 13 lists this hierarchy as follows:

THOSE IN A QUALIFYING RELATIONSHIP TO THE DECEASED PERSON ARE (HIGHEST FIRST):

1.   spouse or partner (including civil or same sex partner)

2.   parent or child (in this context a 'child' can be any age)

3.   brother or sister

4.   grandparent or grandchild

5.   niece or nephew

6.   stepfather or stepmother

7.   half-brother or half-sister

8.   friend of long standing.

HOSPITAL MANAGEMENT "POSSESSION"

A seminal paper [1] outlines relevant legal cases and common law applies viz. Williams vs Williams [1881] Ch D 659 a) the executor of a deceased's will is entitled to take possession of the deceased's body for the purposes of ensuring a suitable burial. b) Further, a person's own directions as to how their body should be disposed of has no weight in law. R vs Stewart [1881] Ch D 659.

It follows from the above that a coroner "owns" the body temporarily pending a Coroner's investigation i.e. Inquest and so holds the power of consent for further actions. If a Coroner is not involved then the consent process i.e. holding of authority for the next action rests with the hierarchy listed above.

Training and research of invasive procedures on the newly dead is not seemingly ethical acceptable though [2].

REFUSAL OF AUTOPSY

The majority of people who refuse an autopsy on children may have reasons that are not religious. Lishimpi *et al* [3] noted that 43% of those who refused autopsy felt that it was a waste of time, 25% wished to proceed to burial and 15% had taboo reasons or concurrence with family issues. Few had religious objections to give consent.

Yet it can be difficult to obtain consent for an autopsy in certain religious faiths [4].

Whilst consent in a matter of death is not usually an issue it is of value to understand the transference of authority that rests within the core of consent.

REFERENCES

[1] Ownership of a corpse". Donald O. Parsons A. Healthcare Risk Reports. Vol. 12. Issue 8. July/August 2006. Page 9

[2] Ethics of Practicing Medical Procedures on Newly Dead and Nearly Dead Patients. Jeffrey T Berger, MD, Fred Rosner, MD, and Eric J Cassell, MD. Journal of General Internal Medicine. 2002 October; 17(10): 774–778. http://www.pubmedcentral.nih.gov/articlerender.fcgi?artid=1495118

[3] Necropsies in African children: consent dilemmas for parents and guardians K Lishimpi, C Chintu, S Lucas, V Mudenda, J Kaluwaji, A Story, D Maswahu, G Bhat, A J Nunn, A Zumla. Archive Diseases in Children 2001;84:463-467 http://adc.bmj.com/cgi/content/abstract/84/6/463

[4] 4.Jewish News of Greater Phoenix online. December 23, 2005/Kislev 22 5766, Volume 58, No. 13 http://www.jewishaz.com/issues/story.mv?051223+medical

CHAPTER 11

Organ Retention / Specimen Retention

Abstract: In the United Kingdom following several hospital scandals the Human Tissue Act of 1961 was updated in 2004. This in the matter of consent lays out specific detail of who can give consent in the living and in the dead.

INTRODUCTION

It will not have gone unnoticed that the removal or organs at a major Children's Hospital in the UK (Alder Hey) ended in a scandal in 1999 which was unearthed through a linkage from a previous scandal involving cardiac surgery at another hospital (Bristol) which was officially uncovered in 1995. The subsequent reports, Kennedy (Bristol) and Redfern (Alder Hey) make for damning reading. The Kennedy Report on the matter of consent suggested that "The sense is gained that informing parents and gaining their consent to treatment was regarded as something of a chore by the surgeons" and "That being so, the sharing of information should be a process. There must be time to take in what has been said by the clinicians, to reflect on it and to raise questions" and "Patients are entitled to know what experience the surgeon or clinician has before giving consent" [1].

The Redfern Report [2] revealed that "Some clinicians applied the threat of a Coroner's post mortem examination to obtain consent to a hospital post mortem examination..... any organs such as the heart or brain which had to be fixed before they could be examined, necessarily meant that not only were they usually retained without consent.... ignoring written consents to limited post mortem examination". One recommendation from this report may not yet have fully penetrated the NHS viz. "The Department of Health, the Royal Colleges and medical schools shall provide training for all those involved in obtaining fully informed consent". A complete chapter (11) is devoted to consent and death (pages 21 - 27).

The legislation in place then was the Human Tissue Act 1961 and as a consequence of the recommendations of the Redfern Report this Act was overhauled to become the Human Tissue Act 2004.

THE HUMAN TISSUE ACT 2004 AND CONSENT [3]

In the matter of consent the Act refers to other issues previously discussed *vis a vis* capacity and children and parental responsibility as well as adults in the matter of the retention of human tissue and the dead body and its purpose for events other than burial or cremation. An offence may occur if the codes and principles within the Act are not adhered to. However, the authority has published a code of practice in consent and human tissue:

The Human Tissue Authority was set up in 2005 under the auspices of the Human Tissue Act 2004 and covers the UK except Scotland which comes under its own jurisdiction. Part of the

Jeffrey C. McILwain

HTA role is to provide codes of conduct which they have done in consent [4] with model post mortem consent forms [5]. The code on consent should be read in conjunction with other HTA documentation and codes such as organ donation, post mortem, removal, storage and disposal of human organs and tissue. The code is explicit that anyone who removes, stores or uses human materials must be satisfied that a system of consent is in place if appropriate; even if they do not take consent themselves (sections 13, 15, 16) [Note that "sections" refers to the Code on Consent and not the Human Tissue Act.]

CONSENT AND THE LIVING

Any removal of human tissue requires consent

☑ for diagnosis or research for now or in the future (sections 22, 24).

However, consent is **not** required (section 25) for the following purposes:

☒ clinical audit

☒ education or training

☒ performance assessment

☒ public health monitoring

☒ quality assurance

CONSENT AND THE DECEASED

Consent is required (section 26) if tissue is to be stored after a coroner's post mortem; and if

☑ removed and stored for anatomical examination,

☑ determining the cause of death,

☑ determining a treatment effect,

☑ obtaining information relevant to a person now or at a future time,

☑ public display,

☑ research of human disorders,

☑ transplantation,

☑ clinical audit,

☑ education or training,

☑ performance assessment,

☑ public health monitoring

Consent is **not** required (section 27) for:

☒ a coroner's investigation of a cause of death

☒ the retention of tissue under a coroner's direction

☒ the retention of tissue pending a criminal investigation.

EXCEPTIONS FOR RESEARCH SPECIFIC CIRCUMSTANCES

(section 28), tissue from a living person may be stored **without** consent if,

☑ the research is ethically approved

☑ the tissue is anonymised.

REFERENCES

[1]   Kennedy   Report   at   bristol-inquiry.org.uk.   final   report.   http://www.bristol-inquiry.org.uk/final_report/rpt_print.htm

[2]   Redfern Report at rlcinquiry.org.uk http://www.rlcinquiry.org.uk/

[3]   Office of Public Sector Information. You are here: Home. Legislation. UK. Acts. Public Acts 2004. Human Tissue Act 2004 (c. 30) http://www.opsi.gov.uk/acts/acts2004/20040030.htm

[4]   Human Tissue Authority. hta.gov.uk. guidance. Codes of Practice. Code of Practice 1: Consent.   http://www.hta.gov.uk/_db/_documents/2006-07-04_Approved_by_Parliament_-_Code_of_Practice_1_-_Consent.pdf

[5]   Human   Tissue   Authority.   hta.gov.uk.   guidance.   Model   consent   forms. http://www.hta.gov.uk/guidance/model_consent_forms.cfm

CHAPTER 12

Human Tissue – Who can give Consent?

Abstract: Whilst it is usual to understand who can give consent in the living, in the matter of death the Human Tissue Act 2004 UK specifies the only hierarchy of who may give consent in death.

THE LIVING

The Living – with Capacity

Only that adult person themselves can give consent although should there be any residual tissue left over after diagnostic purposes the procedure consent form should reflect this, (sections 33, 34). For children the Act defines a child as being a person less than age eighteen years of age. The previous advice of capacity and parental responsibility apply with the equivalence of before (sections 41 - 44).

The Living – with NO Capacity

The use or storage of tissue for those lacking capacity is unlawful **unless** (sections 37 -40)

- ☑ the person acting on behalf of the patient's best interests is assured that the purposes of the tissue may be relevant to another person, now or in the future, or for transplantation.

- ☑ The tissue usage forms part of an approved clinical research programme that specifies actions to be undertaken by those who lack capacity.

- ☑ There is compliance with any appropriate section of the Mental Capacity Act 2005.

FOR THE DECEASED

Adults

If an adult makes a pre-death statement of consent concerning tissue then that remains valid post mortem for which the family or those close to the deceased have no right to veto. For body donation or public display then this requires explicit consent in writing or documented oral, (sections 45 - 47) although no next of kin can give their new consent on behalf of the deceased for anatomical or public display purposes. The hierarchy of nominated representatives for the deceased with whom discussion may occur are given as follows (sections 53 - 59) with the highest first:

1. spouse or partner (including civil or same sex partner)

2. parent or child (in this context a 'child' can be any age)

3. brother or sister

4. grandparent or grandchild

5. niece or nephew

6. stepfather or stepmother

7. half-brother or half-sister

8. friend of long standing.

However, a person within the hierarchy may decline and if the supposed hierarchical person is not available in the time available then a descent down the list is valid. The nominated representative has authority to give consent which cannot be overridden by others. The declaration of a nominated representative is made under the provisions of the Human Tissue Act and must be an adult. The declaration is made pre-mortem and may be in writing with a witness signature or orally in front of two witnesses who will attest to it, [section 4 (1) - (10) of the Act].

Child

A pre-mortem decision remains valid as it does for an adult. If a child cannot make a decision then the responsibility lies with a person with parental responsibility and failing that the hierarchy listed above provided that person is an adult.

Fetal-Maternal Tissue Consent Issues

The Act does not distinguish between fetal tissue and other tissue and regards such tissue as belonging to the mother. A fetus becomes a baby i.e. a living person when any part has been delivered even if cord attached and even if not breathing.

The Code of Practice – Consent gives further advice from section 67 onwards. The advice is in keeping with the general advice already given prior in this book.

CHAPTER 13

Mental Health Patients and Consent

Abstract: Mental health has some very specific requirements that pertain to mental health consent matters and mental illness treatment as well as in the aspect of capacity. This is a specialised field and requires specific knowledge from trained clinicians in the field.

INTRODUCTION

The development of consent aligned with capacity and autonomy comes predominantly from the filed of psychiatry and the professional interactions between clinicians and clients / patients. Landmark cases such as Re:C, have helped formulate the common law position within a framework of ethical principles. Mental Health law is very complex and particular issues pertaining to mental health remain dynamic in law with evolving case law in a rapid manner. Issues that are not simple require the expertise of clinicians and lawyers familiar in the field and current and proposed legislation. There are numerous textbooks and journals devoted to the subject of the application of mental health legislation and its sequelae that readers requiring more in-depth knowledge should consult.

The Mental Health Act 2007 is downloadable [1] from the Office of Public Sector Information. This Act makes reference to the circumstances by which consent applies to mental disorder. Including the use of two signatories and for Electroconvulsive Therapy [page 18 27 - 58A (3) (b) (c)]. Interestingly page 20 28 Section 27: supplemental. (10) the following clause is to be inserted in the Mental Capacity Act viz. In section 28 of the Mental Capacity Act 2005 (c. 9) (Mental Health Act matters), after subsection (1) insert— "(1A) Subsection (1) does not apply in relation to any form of treatment to which section 58A of that Act (electro-convulsive therapy, etc.) applies if the patient comes within subsection (7) of that section (informal patient under 18 who cannot give consent)." This introduces the age of consent for this mental health treatment to be age 18 and not the Gillick competency age of circa 16 although informal treatments and patient aged 16 to 17 is addressed [page 47 section 43] and whilst capacity at this age is accepted a refusal may be countermanded by a person with parental responsibility. Consent can be withdrawn if one sector of treatment has been completed and a subsequent sector is to be started. For immediate treatments within the management of a mental health disorder the patient can consent or an advocate or the Court of protection. [Page 34. 64B Adult community patients. (3) (b) (i) (ii)].

Adults who lack capacity: It is worth quoting directly from the Act as the "rules of engagement" are clearly stated:

"64D Adult community patients lacking capacity. Page 36.

1.   A person is authorised to give relevant treatment to a patient as mentioned in section 64C(2)(c) above if the conditions in subsections (2) to (6) below are met.

2. The first condition is that, before giving the treatment, the person takes reasonable steps to establish whether the patient lacks capacity to consent to the treatment.

3. The second condition is that, when giving the treatment, he reasonably believes that the patient lacks capacity to consent to it.

4. The third condition is that— (a) he has no reason to believe that the patient objects to being given the treatment; or (b) he does have reason to believe that the patient so objects, but it is not necessary to use force against the patient in order to give the treatment.

5. The fourth condition is that— (a) he is the person in charge of the treatment and an approved clinician; or (b) the treatment is given under the direction of that clinician.

6. The fifth condition is that giving the treatment does not conflict with— (a) an advance decision which he is satisfied is valid and applicable; or (b) a decision made by a donee or deputy or the Court of Protection." The issue of children and a lack of capacity are also covered however this area will likely remain contentious as are emergency situations whereby the patient lacks capacity and life preservation or life saving is an apparent necessity [page 37 section 34G].

As in all matters of new legislation clinicians should navigate carefully and under peer advisement as to the interpretation and application of the principles and specifics of the Act.

REFERENCE

[1] the Office of Public Sector Information Home. Legislation. UK. Acts. Public Acts 2007 Mental Health Act 2007 (c. 12). http://www.opsi.gov.uk/acts/acts2007/pdf/ukpga_20070012_en.pdf

CHAPTER 14

Clinical Recordings Including Photography and Images

Abstract: It is not unusual for recordings to be made of clinical matters for the benefit of future audit of care or teaching. Within a digital age the matter of consent is of even more importance as to the capture and storage of such images and their usage thereof.

INTRODUCTION

It has been, and is, common practice to record images of patients for educational, archive or audit purposes. Often such images are used to compare pre-operative and post-operative findings particularly in the surgical disciplines using reconstructive procedures, or, for monitoring disease progress. It is even possible to refute a primary negligence case with a secondary acquisition of evidence viz. a woman had a laparoscopic sterilisation and became pregnant. The issue was "were the clips properly in the correct place on the Fallopian tubes"? No one could answer the question with true evidence without a second procedure which would be deemed inappropriate. However, she did have a second laparoscopic procedure for another reason at another institution and a wise second surgeon ignorant of the primary allegation photographed the clips in situ and so refuted the case indirectly though photographic evidence. The idea that "A picture paints a thousand words" The first time a form of the phrase appears in print is in James Kirke Paulding's *New Mirror for Travellers*, 1828: "A look, which said as plainly as a thousand words." The notion that a visual image is better than a written description has ensured that medical photography is a discipline in its own right for the recording of images for future clinical, audit or legal use.

The Institute of Medical Illustrators has published guidance and a code of conduct that explains most issues for its members [1]. As is usual a primary issue is obtaining consent both for usage and storage of clinical images for professional or educational use. The GMC gives guidance on this matter [2]

Consent (permission) is **not** required for the following for any purposes:

- ☒ Images taken from pathology slides

- ☒ X-rays

- ☒ Laparoscopic images

- ☒ Images of internal organs

- ☒ Ultrasound images

provided that:

☑ The recordings are anonymised

☑ All identifying marks are removed

However, consent is required for recording of the following subject to the caveats above:

☑ For the assessment and treatment of patients

☑ Hospital autopsy

☑ Whereby the recording forms an integral part of the clinical record

☑ When it is possible the patient may be identifiable

St Elsewhere Hospitals
Patient Consent for Medical Photography

ATTACH PATIENT I.D. LABEL or **PRINT** ALL DETAILS	Title _____ First name(s) _____ Family name _____ of Address _____ Address _____ ___/___/___ Date of birth Sex Patient Registration Number
	CONSULTANT IN CHARGE: _____

PLEASE READ AND COMPLETE THIS FORM CAREFULLY

1 I, *(PRINT NAME)* _____ being the patient/the parent of/person with parental responsibility for/the legal guardian of/legal advocate of, the patient *(delete as appropriate)* referred to above, understand that I have been asked to consent to the photographic or video recording of images of myself/the patient.

2 It has been clearly explained to me by_____
PRINT HEALTHCARE PROFESSIONALS NAME
that any recorded images that I consent to be taken, may be used for the teaching of medical or nursing staff or the teaching of clinical students. The doctor / nurse has explained that they understand the need for confidentiality in these matters.

3 If images stored for use in case sheets alone are to be used for future publication in a recognised medical journal or for research purposes or exhibition purposes the Trust will seek further written consent.

I consent to the photographs / video being used for

Case notes		Teaching & Research		Exhibition		Publication	

MARK EACH BOX AS APPROPRIATE e.g.a ✓ or ✗ or INITIALS

⟹ _____   ___/___/___
   Your Signature   Today's date

HEALTHCARE PROFESSIONAL SECTION

The photographs / images / recordings have been taken by [delete a) or b) as appropriate]

a) The Medical Photography Department and are kept there (Ref:_____)

or, b) _____ and copies **are / are not** (delete as appropriate)
PRINT HEALTHCARE PROFESSIONALS TITLE & NAME
held in the Medical Photography Department (Ref:_____).

> I believe that I have clearly explained the use of recorded, photographic or other images to the patient/parent/guardian/advocate and that I fully understand the need for confidentiality of this material. I have obtained written consent to record images or other audio or visual representation from the patient / parent / guardian / advocate / person with parental responsibility.
>
> NAME: _____   SIGNATURE: _____
> *PRINT* Initials & Family name
>
> DATE: ___/___/___ DEPARTMENT: _____
> *N.B. RECORDED IMAGES MADE BE REQUIRED FOR LEGAL EXAMINATION IN THE FUTURE*

FORM 1. EXAMPLE OF A MEDICAL PHOTOGRAPHY CONSENT FORM

There is no advisory necessity for written consent to be taken and oral consent which is documented in the case record may suffice; however, it is prudent that written consent is taken and filed. Each organisation, in the absence of a nationally agreed consent form format will have, or not, a standard consent form. An example of a Trust consent form is shown as Form 1. retention of the consent form within a Medical Illustration Department ensures that there is control and tagging between the recordings and the patient identifier without creating an excess within the case record. The example given is for photographic purposes and with any documentation must be subject to review.

In an emergency or with a temporary capacity loss images may be taken, however, before any usage the patient on regaining capacity must give consent. In a permanent capacity loss then the relevant responsible person within the hierarchy described in tissue donation must be consulted and give permission. During anaesthesia a person may be taken to have a loss of capacity so intra-operation photography or recordings taken ad hoc must have retrospective consent taken.

At any time a patient can withdraw consent and as such this removal of consent will place a restriction on future usage of the recording. Consent giving and removal is dynamic and previous permission granting is not a mark of perpetuity.

Privacy and confidentiality is of paramount importance and so it is important that the patient knows exactly how any recording may be used, or what will happen in the future. Consideration may also be given of how to explain the storage and destruction of any recordings and how long them may be stored for as well as the purpose of the recording.

Consent to use a recording, usually visual, for a journal or text will require further consent as the recording is moving from the privacy of the professional clinical arena and case record to that of the (semi) public arena. It is usual that each publisher will expect explicit consent to publish a recording and will often use a "house style" of consent form or require written consent and release from the patient.

Audio recordings are no different from visual recordings and any such situations require consent as for medical photography. Covert recording is not permissible by any party, nor is it submissible as evidence in a court.

STUDENTS

This can have a consequence within an organisation for clinical students. Healthcare Professionals in training as university undergraduates may undertake audio, or visual, recordings of their engagement with patients as part of their training and education. As members of the university the students and the university may consider that university rules apply. However, such students are visitors to a NHS organisation and are not employees of that organisation, yet the patient belongs to the NHS organisation. It is important that clear direction and advice is laid down between the university and the NHS organisation in the matter of student recording and consent, to ensure a patient's privacy and confidentiality is not unmasked or perverted by the use of recordings of NHS patients on NHS premises by university students. A student make seek consent directly from a patient to record however it would be difficult to be certain that a student is fully aware of their responsibilities in the matter of confidentiality, safe storage, archive, use and disposal of the recording.

The Department of Health advice is encapsulated within their model consent policy section VIII [3].

Consent for photographic or video recordings made for the treatment or assessment of patients care is required and such recordings must be for the purpose of that care including audit. There is no requirement for consent taking provide that;

- ☑ The patient cannot be identified, and

- ☑ The purpose of the recording is for education and training within a clinical setting.

If however the primary reason for recording is for educational, research or publication purposes then consent giving is required.

DIGITAL IMAGES

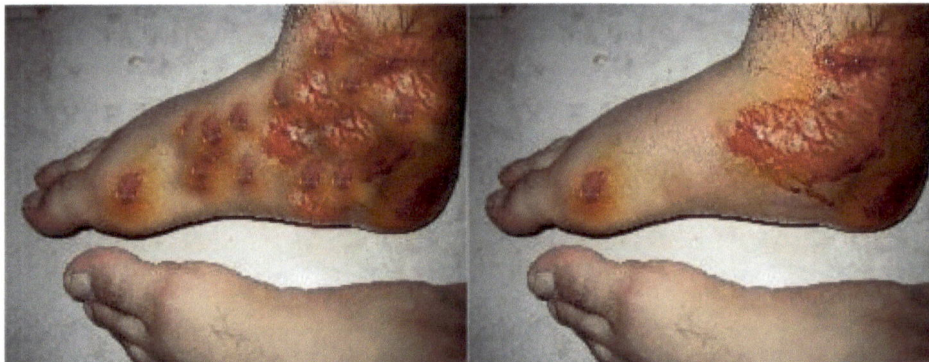

Picture 1. manipulation of a digital photograph with imaging software. Time taken, 6 minutes

In days past in a pre-digital era, images were captured on wet film and the image captured was the effect of a chemical reaction that was permanent. Magnetic style recording was of a similar quality although more destructible. In modern times digital cameras are cheap, made of good quality and are readily available even on mobile telephones. For professional purposes an image is captured after consent is taken, or retrospectively in the incapacitated. However, the public who have access to NHS premises as patients or visitors may carry mobile telephones and capture images without the consent of staff. Such digital images are difficult to ratify or verify when downloaded onto a computer with image manipulating software. The image above (Picture 1) has been digitally manipulated albeit amateurishly by the author, but within 6 minutes. The right hand picture is the original and the left hand picture has been altered. In this case the image on the left displays a more grave injury than first captured. Depending upon which image is taken to be the truth may depend upon the degree of assessment in a court of law and what image is put forward. Whilst the right image may have had consent attached the left will not and so tagging consent to an image or recording made is of supreme importance if digital techniques are used, rather than "wet film" technology.

REFERENCES

[1]   Institute of Medical Illustrators. Home. Law and Ethics. http://www.imi.org.uk/lawethics.htm and http://www.imi.org.uk/code.pdf

[2]   General Medical Council. gmc-uk.org. Home. Guidance on good practice. List of ethical guidance Making and using audio and visual recordings of patients http://www.gmc-uk.org/guidance/current/library/making_audiovisual.asp

[3]   Department of Health. www.dh.gov.uk policy and guidance. Health topics. Consent. Consent key documents. Guidance for clinicians. Download model consent policy in rich text. http://www.dh.gov.uk/prod_consum_dh/idcplg?IdcService=GET_FILE&dID=15623&Rendition=Web

CHAPTER 15

Data Protection / Confidentiality

Abstract: As within any storage of information or sharing, the matter of confidentiality of such information is paramount and probably subject to statute law.

INTRODUCTION

For information to be disclosed may require the consent of the patient. The Department of Health has published a Code of Practice in 2003 for the NHS [1]. In particular information that can identify a patient or their personal circumstances cannot be released without the consent of the patient unless it is of significant public information or there is legal justification to do so, whereas, anonymised information is not regarded as confidential, nor is consent required for audit or record validation. If it is required that information must be communicated between Healthcare Professionals then the patient must give their consent either implied or expressly. If a patient does not wish to have information sharing in healthcare matters they should be advised of the risks that may entail if a secondary person is not privy to all relevant information. If the information is not for healthcare matters then the custodian of the information must ensure that the patient is made fully aware of the circumstances and so give their consent for that purpose. As in other forms of consent the patient has the right to withhold consent unless a significant public reason or legal reason justifies disclosure of information.

For young people aged 16 to 18 they are presumed to have an ability to consent for treatment as before and so are presumed to have an ability to withhold consent for disclosure or approval. Under age 16 the test is as before decision making ability and whether the best interests are served. So a child under 16 may give approval but not withhold consent and the matter of a person with parental responsibility applies. However, if the matter is of a life saving nature then a child's refusal may be overtaken by a person with parental responsibility.

If capacity has been lost by the patient the usual rules of determining best interests and consulting with those who know the patient are to be observed with any disclosure being pertinent to the clinical matter.

In all circumstances the rationale and reasons for disclosure must be conveyed to the patient or whoever acts on their behalf including future confidentiality. Consent remains a requirement under the 1998 Data Protection Act in particular consent is primarily mentioned in Schedules 2 & 3 page 10 [2]. The Health and Social Care Act of 2001 also applies [3].

When dealing with the medial healthcare staff are bound by a duty of care in confidentiality and so to make a comment requires the patient's explicit consent. Any disclosure without consent for "the public interest" must be of an exceptional nature of exceptional public interest, unless that information has already been legitimately placed in the public domain and is factually correct. For full disclosure of a clinical record to a solicitor a full consent disclosure is required. If consent is not forthcoming then a court order or particular public interest can be applied.

In NHS organisations the information governance / confidentiality person is usually a senior clinician and called a Caldicott Guardian [4].

REFERENCES

[1]   Department of Health. Policy and Guidance. Information Policy. Patient confidentiality and access to records. Confidentiality NHS Code of practice http://www.dh.gov.uk/en/Publicationsandstatistics/Publications/PublicationsPolicyAndGuidance/DH_4069253

[2]   2 Office of Public Sector Information Home. Legislation. UK. Acts. Public Acts 1998 Data Protection Act 1998 (c. 29) http://www.opsi.gov.uk/ACTS/acts1998/ukpga_19980029_en_10#sch2

[3]   Office of Public Sector Information Home. Legislation. UK. Acts. Public Acts 2001. Health and Social Care Act 2001 (c. 15) http://www.opsi.gov.uk/acts/acts2001/20010015.htm

[4]   Department of Health. Policy and Guidance. Information Policy. Patient confidentiality and access to records. NHS Caldicott Guardians. The Caldicott Guardian Manual 2006. http://www.dh.gov.uk/en/Publicationsandstatistics/Publications/PublicationsPolicyAndGuidance/DH_062722

CHAPTER 16

Consent and Governance

Abstract: Prior to the more corporate approach to health services it was taken to be the case that consent was a matter between a clinician and a patient. However, today there is more and more inspection and regulation of an organisation's approach to consent taking. This includes the formal details as laid out by regulatory and licensing bodies. By the nature of a public service such aspects of inspection may change more frequently than that of ethics or law pertaining to consent.

CONSENT DELIVERY AND MONITORING

Consent is usually taken to be a private clinical matter between a clinician and a patient. However, the corporate response to the quality of consent taking is a matter for various healthcare inspectorates within the NHS. It is a regarded practice that consent taking should be a regular audited feature of NHS organisations. The NHS Litigation Authority (NHSLA) is responsible for litigation within NHS organisations. It is a special health authority and its website is http://www.nhsla.com/home.htm. From the removal of Crown Immunity the NHSLA has taken over the role of clinical negligence claims within the NHS and third party liability claims. Previously doctors were defended in a clinical negligence claim solely by their Medical Defence Organisation (MDO) even for NHS claims. The NHSLA raises premiums from NHS organisations on an equitable basis proportionate to the clinical services provided e.g. general plus maternity, or Primary Care or Ambulance Trusts or Mental Health Trusts. The annual premium for a Trust can be amended according to the quality of its risk management systems. The scheme that governs this is called the Clinical Negligence Scheme for Trusts (CNST) which is subcontracted to a world wide risk management company Det Norske Veritas (DNV) who set standards in partnership with NHSLA. The scheme for organisations entails 3 levels of risk management achievement from level 1 through to level 3 with each level attracting a 10% discount in premiums which may equate to £250 000 a year per level of achievement. Level 1 is basic and concerns policies in place within an organisation, whilst level 2 is about the policy in action and level 3 how well the policy and system at level 2 is embedded and active within the organisation. The standards are to be found in the risk management area and then linking to CNST standards http://www.nhsla.com/RiskManagement/CnstStandards/ .The general (General secondary Care Trust) standards have 50 sections divided into 5 standards each with 10 criteria, each with a level 1, 2 or 3 level of achievement of which consent is standard 4 criterion 3. The minimum standards for a level 1 document pass is process for obtaining consent

1. process for obtaining consent

2. process for recording consent

3. staff who are not capable of performing the procedure but are authorised to obtain consent

4.   generic training on the consent process

5.   procedure-specific training on consent for staff to whom the consent process is delegated and who are not capable of performing the procedure

6.   process for monitoring the effectiveness of all of the above

For level 2, as level 1 relating to ensuring there is compliance to the policy in level 1 and

1.   staff who are not capable of performing the procedure but are authorised to obtain consent

2.   procedure-specific training on consent for staff to whom the consent process is delegated and who are not capable of performing the procedure.

For level 3, as level 2 and there is monitoring of the compliance

1.   staff who are not capable of performing the procedure but are authorised to obtain consent.

2.   procedure-specific training on consent for staff to whom the consent process is delegated and who are not capable of performing the procedure.

Where the monitoring has identified deficiencies, there must be evidence that recommendations and action plans have been developed and changes implemented accordingly.

There are no parallel standards around consent in Maternity Units / Trusts nor Mental Health and Learning Disability Trusts.

In the matter of the external audit / assessment of risk management standards for acute and primary care Trusts the assessment of the organisation's consent processes constitutes 1 of the 50 domains and so contributes towards 2% of the final assessment pass mark. This means that all the constituent components of the organisation's consent system i.e. consent policy, consent forms, training needs and targets, delegated consent taking, procedure – specific consent training and audit etc must be addressed. A regular (annual) audit of consent forms ensures that an organisation is compliant with monitoring of the use of a consent form by sampling the use of the form to certain agreed criteria. Any deficits arising from the consent audit can then be fed back into the organisation's governance system to be addressed through the education and training process as required.

For acute Trusts this may be a more simple exercise than for a PCT. In an acute Trust usually the organisation is more cohesive in that all staff are employees of a single organisation. This makes the management and audit of the process easier. Within a PCT there may be a range of dispersed geographical units i.e. individual general practices that effectively function as autonomous businesses under a corporate umbrella. This makes the assessment and corporate control of standardised practice in consent taking more difficult. However as the thrust of political healthcare delivery changes towards more procedures performed in primary care then a traditional approach and standard of consent recording may require harmonisation to ensure compliance with NHSLA standards in consent.

Consider a skin mole from the perspective of that skin mole. In an acute Trust with a strong tradition of formalised systems the mole with it's host (the patient) will be placed in a strong consent environment for it's indicated removal probably under a local anaesthetic and probably using consent form 3 (not for general anaesthetic) with the complete and attendant processes and systems that surround the procedure such as pre-operative assessment and waiting list management. The same mole clinically managed in primary care comes under a more local auspice – i.e. that of the individual general practitioner who may, or may not, feel obligated to follow as formal a route as occurs in acute secondary care. The mole 'consent' may then vary yet the risks etc must remain the same as the procedure is the same. One clinical problem two possible methods and approaches to the clinical management *vis a vis* consent. As procedures decant from secondary care to primary care the consent process must remain universally the same otherwise both patient and the Healthcare Professional may be guilty of a "legal foul".

It should be noted that these standards although fundamental to an organisation's risk appraisal may vary on a biennial or triennial basis according to the conduct set by NHSLA and the subcontracted company.

It is apparent from the NHSLA perspective that whilst consent taking is important at the outset that delegated consent taking is of substantial importance as a running theme through out all 3 levels for acute Trusts and Primary Care Trusts (PCTs). An autonomous and trained practitioner has the right to take consent for procedures that they are competent and knowledgeable in. However, as in any delegation, it is important that the delegator ensures that the delegate (the person to whom authority and responsibility has been delegated to) is acting fully and lawfully on the delegator's behalf. The delegate must be fully conversant with the subject matter. This places a duty upon each - the delegator and the delegate i.e. a duty of care. The delegator must ensure to their own satisfaction that the delegate can perform the role required in a manner required with the information required. The delegate must ensure that they have evidence to show that they can fulfil the role required of them. As in consent between a practitioner and a patient there is once again a transfer of authority, in this case between the delegator and the delegate. To ensure the delegate is competent it is prudent to ensure that there is a competency audit trail and a "signing off" by the delegator as perceiving the delegate "to be deemed competent". By ensuring a record of competency gained the delegate can assure a patient of their provenance and so if faced with the question of "what is your experience of this procedure?" the delegate can truly reflect from their assessment evidence and portfolio rather than a bland statement of "I've seen this procedure 6 times" which actually does not answer the question. Further, such a competency portfolio can build to a competency licence. By reviewing the competency on a regular basis or through audit allows the ability of the delegate to be actively monitored and so enhances the quality of a person acting as a delegate for someone else. An example of a form that can be used is below – Form 1. competency agreement..

DELEGATED CONSENT – MONITORING RECORD
Mark all responses with a ✓ in the appropriate ☐

Is the delegate a Nurse ☐ or a Doctor ☐ or a Therapist ☐?

Is this a primary assessment ☐ or a review / follow up assessment ☐ ?

Delegator's details: *(the person delegating consent taking)* PRINT

FAMILY NAME	FIRST NAME
SPECIALITY / DIRECTORATE	**GRADE / TITLE**

Delegate's details: *(the person to who consent taking has been delegated)* PRINT

FAMILY NAME	FIRST NAME
SPECIALITY / DIRECTORATE	**GRADE / TITLE**

LEARNING & ASSESSMENT METHODS USED

DELEGATE		DELEGATOR	
LEARNING METHOD: *tick those which apply*	↓	**ASSESSMENT METHOD:** *tick those which apply* ↓	
Observation		Direct observation	
Discussion with peer		Discussion with delegate	
Text reading		Recognised assessment tool	
Internal Trust course		Group discussion	
External-to-Trust course		Peer discussion	
Recognised learning package		Certification from a course attended	
Direct tuition		Chart review	
Part of a qualification		Audit	
Audit		Other	

In my opinion the person (delegate) named above is competent to perform the taking of consent on my behalf for the procedures listed below. The delegate and I acknowledge that our knowledge must be kept up to date and that this is our duty of care and responsibility; we agree that the knowledge used in consent delegation will be reviewed in an agreed period e.g. 3 years, or sooner, if there is an identified need for update. Expected review date =

_____   _____
Delegator's signature   *date*

CLINICAL PROCEDURE (delegate consent competent)		CLINICAL PROCEDURE (delegate consent competent)	
1.		6.	
2.		7.	
3.		8.	
4.		9.	
5.		10.	
STRIKE-THROUGH UNUSED BOX(S) *e.g.* →			

The Care Quality Commission is responsible for assessing quality standards in care and health [1] and has certain outcome standards for their inspections of care and health organisations including. Outcome 2 : Consent to care and treatment: People using the service:- Where they are able, give valid consent to the examination, care, treatment and support they receive. - Understand and know how to change any decisions about examination, care, treatment and support that has been previously agreed. - Have systems in place to gain and review consent from people who use services, and act on them. It is not yet apparent how this aligns with NHSLA standards.

REGULATORY CHANGES

In July 2010 the British Government has proposed substantial changes to NHS healthcare delivery in England with the proposed dissolution of Primary Care Trusts. The consequences from the perspective of the assessment of consenting practice in primary care, amongst other matters, remains unclear.

INFORMATION VERIFICATION

It is taken as good practice that lay people should be involved in the development and ratification of information being imparted as part of clinical information. It is traditional custom and practice that professionals seek out information to apply to their information giving process. Often this task may be delegated to someone with less experience of the senior clinician and so a lack of control into the sourcing of the information and its quality may arise. Often the development of patient information includes both a brief description of the procedure (although often lacking a full layout of the seven principles of patient information outlined previously) mixed with other information such as access, visiting times, what to bring etc. This dilutes the procedure "message". Further a professional may import such consent information from another source but has not ensured its veracity or relevance presuming that the publication of such information is both pertinent and reliable, particularly if the information is deemed to be from a "superior" source. However, each individual organisation is responsible for ensuring that information used by that organisation is strong and relevant and should not presume that an imported source of information is of sufficient quality. To enable such ratification to take place the concept of a Patient Information Group should be considered. This helps to ensure that imported information is relevant to the organisation and its local health community. There are instances of professionals creating information that does not stand up to scrutiny when assessed for example on readability grounds. If lay people without the duress of a proposed procedure cannot understand a procedure's description then there is little hope for a patient who may feel forced to a) make a choice about having the procedure or not and b) make their mind up in a short period of time, to go on a waiting list, or, risk losing or deferring that position. It is prudent therefore that organisation's have a system or committee or group to ratify imported information clinical and non-clinical to ensure that the organisation can stand over its information. Further, this helps clinicians ensure that they are part of the corporate delivery rather than acting fully free which may place themselves at risk of defending information that they have imported but is not truly representative or reflective of their skills or practice.

INFORMATION GOVERNANCE

Following on from the above it is important that an accessible site is available to obtain information or download it from a registered and approved Website. A medical negligence claim can begin effectively from the date of knowledge i.e. the date that harm was determined and a defendant identified. This may mean that a claim for medical negligence can arise some time after the apparent occurrence of the incident. Further, in the matter of a child in particular a brain damaged child the time limit may effectively be up to birthday age of 21. For an adult there is a limitation to the date a claim can be made which is 3 years from the identification of the harm and the defendant although there may be no time limit if the adult is brain damaged and has lost capacity. Once the harm is identified then any reference around consent and patient information will relate to the time of the harm's occurrence. This means that all clinical information that is imparted must be archived as pertinent to the time of the harm.

DIRECT WAITING LIST ACCESS

Although not a common occurrence it is foreseeable that a rapid solution to patients having to wait is direct access from a primary care assessment to a secondary care service in a different organisation. The difficulty arises on who is deemed to a) be the recommending clinician and b) the person with ultimate charge for the care of the patient. In the BMA consent tool kit 2007 *q.v.* it is stated that *"The BMA considers that the doctor who recommends that the patient should undergo the intervention should have responsibility for providing an explanation to the patient and obtaining his or her consent. In a hospital setting this will normally be the senior clinician."* In a direct access service to a waiting list then the recommending doctor would be that in the primary care service. Yet, the technical person with charge over the patient's actual procedure would be within the 'hospital' setting. The parallel to this dilemma occurs already with screening services and investigative procedures. If one considers that the doctor who is before the patient is the one with most knowledge of that patient they may be considered duty bound to advise the patient about the procedure before the patient embarks upon it. It cannot be presumed that a patient who is told that "you need an investigation" i.e. an invasive procedure is fully informed or knowledgeable about that procedure particularly if the referring doctor is not either and in particular if that procedure carries frequent or significant risks. It is prudent to suggest that the doctor or clinician performing that invasive clinical procedure should take the consent for that procedure. However, this will require pre-procedural time and a clear knowledge of pertinent facts surrounding the patient's personal medical history. The situation may be further compounded if the referring doctor in the primary care service is availing themselves of a NHS organisation that they are contracted to use. Managing the risk boundaries between organisations can be fraught and in the matter of consent even more so as regards liability and a duty of care [3].

REFERENCES

[1]   The   Care   Quality   Commission.   Outcome   standards. http://www.cqc.org.uk/yourviews/feedbackfromlocalgroups/outcomes.cfm

[2]   Exploring the boundaries of risk within and between NHS organisations. McILwain J.C. Health Care Risk Report. 2006.vol 12 issue 6. Page 12-13

CHAPTER 17

Stretch Yourself: Some Consent Scenarios

Abstract: It is useful to discuss scenarios that are real or construed to test one's understanding and so 30 scenarios are given for enlightenment based upon the text of founding principles.

CONSENT CLUB

Like a journal club there is a place to consider forming a professionally lead "Consent Club" within a clinical department or organisation. Such a club meeting regularly and involving all clinicians of all seniority can easily look at consent. By testing scenarios based upon age, capacity, seniority of clinician set against law, ethics and risk management principles can allow both education and development of solutions to thorny consent issues. By role playing (under a referee i.e. chairperson as consent issues can become quite heated when ethics and law abut) as Medical Director, Senior Doctor or Nurse or as trainee then the issues that arise can settle knowledge levels and attain a more even playing field of ability and performance. Further, as the group develops it's skills then potential issues of consent can be addressed. In this way the forum can allow difficult consent issues to be discussed in advance and professional decisions made and recorded a kind of Bolam-Test-in Advance. This can help ensure that an individual clinician with a difficult consent issue has the support and debate of their colleagues and help arrive at a decision that is anchored in knowledge and experience across many specialities and so pertinent to the individual clinical care that the patient may require. By taking minutes of such meetings and decisions then there is justifiable advance peer reasoning should a complaint or allegation of negligence arise.

SCENARIOS

What follows is a list of simple or even thorny scenarios that doctors and nurses have, or may face. No answers are given as consent issues are not so simple otherwise there would be no texts on the subject and no lawyers in business. The standalone question or scenario is to encourage thinking around consent rather than an off-the-shelf easy answer. Two clinicians faced with the same consent issue may arrive at different answers which depend as much upon the patient and their decision as it does upon the clinician's perspective. There are no "right answers" in the mathematical sense of 'A' is correct and so 'B' by default is not, but perhaps there are wrong answers, or wrong ways of going about consent or problem solving. Individuals may find some solutions within the text and some will lie outside the text as they are posed dilemmas that do not lend themselves to simple scrutiny. In each case the "pupil" should respond to the scenario from the perspective of law, ethics and risk intertwined rather than a pure legal or pure ethics or pure risk perspective.

Each posed scenario should be concluded by asking yourself **"what do you do now / next?"**

Scenario 1   The daughter of an elderly patient says that she will sign her mother's consent form for knee replacement, as her mother cannot come to the hospital to sign it being restricted in her movement.

Scenario 2 A 10 year old child is scheduled for a routine tonsillectomy. The father, unmarried, says that he will sign the consent form as the child's mother cannot get time off work and it will make everyone's life easier now that he is actually here.

Scenario 3 A 10 year old child is scheduled for a routine tonsillectomy. The grandfather says that he will sign the consent form as the child's mother cannot get time off work and he looks after the child 3 days a week so knows all about the child.

Scenario 4 John is 21 and has severe learning disability. He needs an elective circumcision. The consultant in charge of John's surgery says to the registrar that the relatives can come in and sign the consent form on John's behalf.

Scenario 5 Mary is 17 living on her own and needs a rapidly enlarging mole removed from her leg. She refuses to have an operation.

Scenario 6 Sarah is 16 and her child Mark aged 6 months needs a circumcision. Sarah refuses surgery, but Mark's father Billy also aged 16 says that he will sign the consent form. The parents are not married.

Scenario 7 Simon is 17 and needs a defunctioning colostomy. Simon's parents are devout Jehovah's Witnesses and forbid Simon to have blood products should he haemorrhage. Simon is uncertain if he wants the operation.

Scenario 8 Mary aged 82 has a fractured neck of femur and has waited 3 days for her operation due to staff shortages. Mary has severe dementia. Her husband Maurice cares for her. She comes to theatre but no consent form has been signed.

Scenario 9 In a busy outpatient's clinic Mr Cutoff, the consultant surgeon declares that Mr Inpain (a patient) needs a haemorrhoidectomy and that the consent form can be completed in the pre-operative clinic by the pre-operative clinic staff.

Scenario 10   You are a clinical specialist and fully trained and competent in five defined surgical procedures. Mr Cutoff has deemed you competent for these five procedures. Mr Inpain (a patient) needs a haemorrhoidectomy and Mr Cutoff says that you can take the consent for the haemorrhoidectomy as "you know the drill" even though this is not one of the five procedures you are deemed competent in.

Scenario 11   Miss Confused is a patient who has been admitted under the Mental Health Act for her mental illness of schizophrenia. She develops a serious infection in her leg. She is advised by the psychiatric staff that she needs surgery as in debridement and possible amputation, Miss Confused is adamant that she does not want surgery even though she fully understands the consequences. She believes that she must die without ever having an operation on her legs. Mr Cutoff the surgeon decides that the leg must come off and tells the staff that they must consent the patient, to save her life as it is in her best interests. He instructs the staff to consent the patient for amputation surgery.

Scenario 12   You are a clinical specialist and fully trained and competent in five surgical procedures. Mr Cutoff has deemed you competent for these five procedures. Mr Inpain (a patient) needs an operation that is not in your five procedures, but is quite similar to one of them. Mr Cutoff says that you can take the consent for the procedure as it so similar to the five others you know about.

Scenario 13   Cybil has lived with her partner Maud for 25 years in a relationship. Cybil develops a femoral hernia that is at risk of strangulation if left untreated. Cybil regards Maud as her "next of kin". Whilst waiting to be admitted Cybil develops a stroke (Cerebro-Vascular Accident) and loses the power of communication but indicates to her GP that she wishes Maud to act on her behalf in all things clinical. Cybil is due for surgery and Maud is consulted by the medical team as regards consent. However, Cybil's son James whom she has not seen nor heard off for 15 years arrives from Australia and refuses to let Cybil have her operation for her hernia.

Scenario 14   Mrs 'X' has a lesion on her cervix that requires to be removed under a general anaesthetic. During the procedure Dr 'Z' a trainee from a foreign country visiting as a registered clinical fellow in the gynaecological department notices a bleeding and odd shaped skin lesion on the inside thigh of the patient and asks the scrub nurse for a scalpel in order to remove it as it may be a cancer.

Scenario 15   Miss 'G' is a woman who requires a hysterectomy for fibroids, she is aged 60. The registrar from another country proceeds to perform the operation and then starts to remove the ovaries as "that is what standard practice in my own country is".

Scenario 16   Mr 'V' aged 34 has decided he needs a vasectomy for contraceptive purposes. His partner says she will also sign the consent form as well.

Scenario 17   Mr 'J' is a fit clear minded 90 year old who served in the Army for many years. He respects doctors. He would benefit from a knee replacement. You begin to explain to him the procedure. He stops you and says "Just do whatever you think is best doctor, I trust your judgement".

Scenario 18   Cheryl is 19 and a single mum. Ryan her 2 year old child requires corrective surgery on a squint. Ryan's father (Dave) left the family 20 months ago and has never been heard of since and never married Cheryl. Ryan arrives at the ward for his operation, however, Dave who is an orderly on this ward, demands that the operation does not go ahead as he is Ryan's father and "knows his rights".

Scenario 19   Liz and Suzanne have been in a stable relationship for 10 years and in a civil partnership for 2 years. They want a child and Liz becomes pregnant through a friend. At 3 months gestation Liz wants an abortion but Suzanne objects. The friend has since died in an accident.

Scenario 20   Brian and Mark are in a civil partnership and have adopted a 2 year old child. The child needs an elective hernia operation. Brian agrees and is willing to consent but Mark disagrees and refuses to give consent.

Scenario 21   Mary has a suspected skin lesion on her eyelid and beside her mouth. She is scheduled to have these lesions removed under local anaesthetic at the local plastic surgery department. Dr 'P' is a visiting doctor from another country and during the procedure starts to take photographs of Mary's face of the procedure to remove the lesions to add to his collection of photographs.

Scenario 22   James is an elderly man who dies in hospital. He was given a drug that is new to the department although it is licensed for the purpose for which it is used. There have been a few reports of this drug having effects that are non-therapeutic but not proven to be life threatening. Dr 'W' reports the case to the coroner who takes jurisdiction. The family however refuse to allow a post mortem as it is against their culture.

Scenario 23   Brian has had part of his face removed for a rhabdomyosarcoma of his orbit and has had a plastic surgery reconstruction of the defect. Brian learns "from a mate" that the specimen of his face has been kept and is mounted in a bottle in the pathology laboratory teaching room without his consent.

Scenario 24   Brenda is scheduled to have an invasive clinical procedure. She has been informed of the risks etc and one risk that does concern her is the risk of infection of the wound as her mother died from septicaemia. She reads on the Internet that at the local hospital where her procedure will be performed that their infection rates after surgery are five times greater than on her information sheet and asks about the "true" rate of infection.

Scenario 25   Andrew visits his GP with a rapidly growing and bleeding wart on his hand. His GP used to be a surgical trainee and tells Andrew that "it is no problem" and that he will arrange for it to be removed at a local clinic where he does some work. He tells Andrew that the nurse will inform of everything he needs to know. An appointment is made for the following week. No information about the procedure is give to Andrew nor is any sent out in the post. The following week the GP asks Andrew at the clinic "is it OK to go ahead then since you are here?" Andrew nods. The skin lesion is removed and is reported as a malignant melanoma with unclear margins.

Scenario 26   Martin is a drug addict and has had several hospital admissions for overdoses. He is admitted to the Emergency Department with another suspected overdose. He waves a piece of paper in the air that he states to be a "Living Will". In this document there is a statement in handwriting that if he (Martin) should ever take another overdose then he refuses to be resuscitated under any circumstance. The piece of paper is signed by Martin and dated one week ago.

Scenario 27   Mr Black is a 67 year old retired man with other medical problems including type 2 diabetes and who develops a cardiac arrhythmia and sent and investigated by a cardiologist. He has several treatment options offered to him, one of which includes an ablation of an aberrant nerve pathway in his heart. Mr Black tells the cardiologist that he wants this procedure and the risks are explained to Mr Black, including the risk of myocardial infarction. Mr Black insists that the procedure must go ahead as he has a cruise booked, and if he has a cardiac arrest then all attempts to resuscitate him must be performed and he must be admitted to an intensive care unit and kept alive. Mr Black has a very strong family history of heart disease. He says he fully gives his consent to be fully resuscitated and his son is a solicitor.

Scenario 28   Alex is 15 and cannot communicate his wishes since he had a brain injury 5 years ago. His mother is his sole carer. Alex develops recurrent nose bleeds that are alarming. He is taken to the local specialist who cannot see a bleeding point but suspects that there is something much further up Alex's nose that requires a procedure to remove, (probably under a general anaesthetic). Alex's mother is distraught and tells the doctor "to do whatever is necessary and she will sign the form".

Scenario 29   Gail is a 5 year old child who puts foreign bodies in her ears. They usually fall out. Gail is hyperactive. She places a bead in her right ear and is sent up to the nurse lead emergency ENT clinic where it is confirmed that there is a bead in the right ear which cannot be removed at clinic and so requires it to be removed under general anaesthetic. Gail is listed from the emergency ENT clinic and scheduled for removal of foreign body from her right ear the following week on Mr Nares's (the consultant) operating list. At operation the consent is noted to be "removal of foreign body form right ear". Mr Nares proceeds with successful removal of the foreign body from the right ear. However he also examines the left ear and performs a myringotomy (incision in the ear drum) and finds fluid (glue ear) in the middle ear and inserts a ventilating tube (grommet). He tells Gail's mother afterwards that in his experience children with glue ear put foreign bodies in their ears as the glue ear disturbs them and that is likely why Gail is hyperactive. Gail's mother only consented to the removal of the foreign body.

Scenario 30   Peter is a highly skilled joiner and restores marquetry on antique tables and furniture. He is tired all the time and attends his GP surgery. His GP orders routine blood tests to be performed by the practice nurse. At the blood session the nurse is a trainee attending for venepuncture training under the supervision of the practice nurse. After 4 attempts the trainee nurse succeeds in getting some blood from the forearm but inadvertently stabs the ulnar nerve leaving Peter with numbness down his hand for 8 weeks and so is unable to work.

INDEX

A

Advance statements, 45

Autonomy, 6

B

Best Interests, 7

C

Capacity, 9

Clinical images, 63

Clinical research, 48

Communication difficulty and patients, 41

Consent delivery and monitoring, 70

Consent expressions, 13

Consent Forms, 27

Coroner and consent, 53

D

Delegating Consent, 36

Discomforts, 15

Doctors in Training, 38

Doctors taking consent, 23

Duration, 29

Duty of care, 2

E

Elective procedures, 33

Emergency situations, 33

www.ingramcontent.com/pod-product-compliance
Lightning Source LLC
Chambersburg PA
CBHW041721210326
41598CB00007B/735